THE RITUAL

CW01501979

WHY THIS BOOK?

I am living in a time of wonders.

Beliefs about the limits of human potential are changing. Fifty years ago when I was a young man I doubt if I would have had the ability to write this book. I could not have worked out for myself the miracle of what it is to be human, the unlimited nature of our gifts, the power that is within each of us to take control of our lives, our health, the rate at which we age, indeed the extent to which we engage with the ageing process.

I have never written a book. Do not profess to holding any credentials that merit my recognition as a writer, and I am certainly not an academic, but I do believe I have information that is worth sharing. I have changed my life, improved my health, and dramatically altered my expectations as to how I will live out the rest of my existence, by creation and performance of a simple Ritual.

It is a fact that each one of us has a hand to play in how old we become. Not in our chronological age, but in how we present, how aged we seem, in the ability and faculty we retain and in our continuing 'youthfulness' and the extent of our decrepitude.

It is time to change perspective, to recognise that each and every one of us is involved and participant in the process of our ageing. We are not merely observers. Ageing is not some inexorable and dominant force upon our life. We age ourselves, just as we choose a car, or choose a house, we choose if we are to age or to remain vital and in good health.

The purpose of this book is to introduce you to a ritual. My Ritual. My invented regime that is a mental, spiritual and therapeutic workout performed every day.

The Ritual I have created, heals, rejuvenates, maintains and changes, everything. Not only our mindset, although that will be the first thing to alter, but our being, how we present, the energy we have, how we appear, the state we are in.

ORIGINS OF THE RITUAL

It is astonishing to write that such a positive therapy as the Ritual was born out of cynicism and doubt but that is the fact.

I no longer believed in those dispensing my good health. I do not mean that I doubted the sincerity or commitment of the doctors and nurses who had trained to be part of a national health provision service. I doubted the service itself. I doubted that such a vast machine as a national health provider could really determine what was wrong with me when I was ill and fix it. I doubted the sincerity of the drug manufacturers. How do they know their drugs will suit me? Their drugs are trialled but the trial results are not published. We have no league table of successful pills. We have no chart identifying the number of us who have suffered side effects, or even more significantly, information about deaths in which use of a particular drug may be implicated.

Even more to the point we have no information on the league table of 'earners', the medicines the companies would like to persuade the medical profession to prescribe, because they deliver huge profit margins.

I may be an ordinary man without power or voice but I would like to know. I would like to know also about

THE RITUAL

HOW TO LIVE LONGER,
LOOK YOUNGER,
BE HEALTHIER

ROBERT GLYN JONES

Published by **Robert Glyn Jones Publishing**

Copyright Robert Glyn Jones©2014

ISBN: 978-0-9932342-0-0

'all truth passes through three stages. First, it is ridiculed. Second, it is violently opposed. Third, it is accepted as being self evident.'
Arthur Schopenhauer.
19th century German philosopher.

CONTENTS

Introduction   Foreward ix

Chapter 1   Belief..1

Chapter 2   The Power of Placebo 18

Chapter 3   Triggers 50

Chapter 4   Building Blocks 75

Chapter 5   The Ritual Process 117

Chapter 6   The Ritual for the Lymph System 133

Chapter 7   The Ritual Exercises 145

Chapter 8   The Everyday Facelift...............................164

Chapter 9   The Recumbent Gym 185

Chapter 10   Explanations..216

Chapter 11   Positivity 239

Chapter 12   Miracles..256

Chapter 13   Diet and Lifestyle......................................274

Chapter 14   Other Secrets...294

the less effective medicines the, 'generic substitutes', the ones Health Authorities may want prescribed by every practitioner working for them because they are cheaper to buy? Do they work as well as the big brand guys? Am I allowed to enquire?

Before I invented my Ritual and took back control of my health I felt powerless, anonymous, without any distinguishing characteristic dependent upon my own genetics that made my illness different in nature to everyone else's. Illnesses in mainstream medicine do not vary. Piles are piles, asthma is asthma, cancer is cancer. Human physiology and biology is known and mapped. If a pill works it works. If a surgical procedure works it works. But what if it doesn't and what if it does when there is no medical or pharmacological reason that it should.

What about the outrageous tendency of human beings to be individuals and ruin everything? Every equation, every scientific test result, defied and contradicted by the idiosyncracies of the 'non average' man and women. How many of us are in that category?

' Non average', ' Idiosyncratic', ' Individual'

Everyone in the world, I suggest, but of course mass medicine cannot cater for that. To keep a giant breathing things have to be streamlined, packaged, organized in to ten minute consultation slots and detailed triage maps of expected action. The ultimate hope and expectation of those administering a national health service, being I presume, that human assessors can be dispensed with and the dispensing of cures standardised to allow computers to take charge. The end point of reform, some administrators vision, of computers ready in every health centre to receive a patient's symptom list.

In the streamlined world of modern medicine you and I as patients are already without voice. Our only responsibility at present is to be ill, to attend with symptoms and let the show unfold, the referrals be made, the scans organized, the diagnosis presented.

We have absolutely no control over the process of our 'cure', and we are not supposed to have. We are supposed to accept whatever diagnosis is handed out and we are supposed to accept whatever pill or potion is given to us to ingest, unquestioningly.

Prior to creation of my Ritual I felt overwhelmed by the vastness and indifference of the health system I was required to interact with and I felt powerless. It struck me that I had handed over control of my 'wellness' to a system that did not even see me. Did not know who I was, beyond the coded patient number I wore on a bracelet on my arm. The preoccupation of those attending me at my last consultation was not my own psyche, or any relevant interaction between my emotions and the illness with which I presented, no, that was far too specific, the medics around me at my last consultation were intent on ensuring the numbers on the paper bracelet on my arm matched the number coded on to my medical records.

I at that moment felt invisible. I realised my health care would always be like this unless I looked elsewhere, outside of conventional medicine, to an alternative therapy, or to myself, to cure any illness I was afflicted by.

I have created a Ritual that delivers my 'wellness'. It is not packaged for anyone else. It is not one size fits all, it is a simple but effective therapy tailored at present to myself that can be adapted by anyone wishing to engage with it to suit their own life. My Ritual is not only for the ill, it is for those already well who wish to remain well.

Who am I, you will ask, that I presume to create a Ritual that can bestow health benefits? Well I am not a trained physician. I have no triage charts of required action or drug reference guide for prescribing. I hold no shares at all in the pharmaceutical industry. I am an ordinary guy, beyond the world of mainstream medicine, excluded from the laboratories of the drug manufacturers; in other words, I am as vulnerable as everyone else.

I am almost 70 years old and I do not want some medic, specialist or so called expert to look at me and decide I am in the last decade or so of my life and therefore any medical complaint or disease I am afflicted by is to be expected. Even worse in the event of my sudden death I do not want any coroner or other medic to sign off my death as understandable or natural, because I have lived more than seventy years.

I want to be treated as an individual and I want everyone reading this book to reclaim his or her individuality and to think differently about ageing and the proclaimed inevitability of degeneration, decline and worsening health, that supposedly comes with age. Lifetimes are extending, we need to think differently about the body we have, what it can do, and how long it can be sustained in a shape that makes life pleasurable rather than an existence.

We are brainwashed into believing decay is our fate and I want to brainwash everyone to think in a different more positive way. I want the first thought of my readers upon waking to be full of hope and anticipation and belief in their own power to intervene in the days and the life that they create.

The barometer of age shifts as we evolve and life gets longer. In Britain today those of 90 can still reliably, I believe, be considered old, those of 80 probably, those of 70, 75, probably not, while those of 60 are suddenly rendered incapable of placing within a category. Those of 60 used to be old but they are certainly not now.

Those who have reached and exceeded the age of 100 are vastly increasing in number. It is not miraculous, or even extraordinary, to have everyone in a care home aged over 95.

Science and evolution is changing the ball game but one thing is lagging behind, the manner in which each of us, individually, adjusts our thinking to recognise we are going to be here for a very long time. For much longer than we ever considered when we were planning our retirement, and certainly for a good deal longer than we anticipated when we were investing in pension plans or ignoring the suggestion that pension investment was a good idea.

When we reach 65, or 67, or 68, or whatever age the government decides is our new retirement age we are likely to have decades ahead of us. This book asks that we address one question. What are we going to do with these years? How are we going to exist?

The convention is to believe our energy for life will deplete as we age, our physical capability will reduce and our mental acuteness will be impaired.

Do you want to believe that?

Do you wish to live for several decades in such a reduced state?

Mainstream medicine does not care. It has the flow charts of treatment decisions, the anatomical diagrams for hip replacements, the pills for diabetes ready and waiting. You can live as you are expected to or you can decide not to give in, not to surrender to expected thinking but to adopt another approach to living the rest of your life. This book will help you. Armed with the information it contains you may begin to see the possibility of caring for yourself before decline sets in.

Without the purchase of this book all the guides and signposts our society creates and hands out to the ready to be elderly would be likely to take you in a very different direction.

The message from the state health providers is that the old are burdensome. High maintenance. Billions of pounds on hip replacements, Alzheimer care, worn out hearts, depression, diabetes, cholesterol pills. The message from the drug companies is that the old are money.

Western society successfully inculcates the belief in millions and millions of pensioners that tidy and small routines are enough to sustain a life after the age of 65.

The whole of society works on the precept that later decades are not for input or contribution but for incarceration in a closed world of flower shows and nine holes of golf.

I simply grew tired of the standard messages, of the negativity and the mass programming of expectations for the aged. I did not want to be part of a mass diagnosis of my future health, I wanted to have some control and to do that I knew I had to get to know myself, to understand what I was made of and how I really worked. It took a lot of time. A lot more time than I would have been allocated by those working in a National Health Service but that was fine. I had the time, and if you do not, do not despair because the information I have gained in the last five years can also change your life.

A few years ago I began to read voraciously, everything I could find, that was to do with health and ageing. I asked questions, rang up important medical men, and I found out the greatest set of facts of my life.

I found out the truth about how to live my life.

The truth, or indeed a whole set of truths, that not only altered my perception of everything I had believed in my life but also fundamentally altered the way that I lived and intended to live and keep living over what I now believe will be health filled decades.

I don't wish to be seen as arrogant in making that prediction. I know I should not tempt fate and I am not. I surrender to this great and magnificent Universe, to any accident, catastrophe or disaster, it may have in store for me, but at the same time I say thank you Universe because I have discovered the true power within it and within myself.

I am the same as every reader reading this book. The only difference between you and I is that I am a little further ahead in my quest for health. I have a few more facts, know a few more things simply as a result of the doubt I possessed that the approach society and my national health service would have me follow towards health was the only route I could take.

This book contains numerous references to academic and medical publications, to websites and institutions, sufficient to lead anyone to all the information that has inspired and helped me to see 'the bigger picture'. I have shared, all I now know, in the hope that by my final chapter every purchaser of this book will be as equipped as I now am to make the transition from aged to elderly, to ancient, a smooth and pain free glide.

A daily dose of my Ritual will help every one to access the health they deserve. I hope by the end of this book your own view of the ageing process and the responsibility we each have to engage with and prevent its often deleterious consequences, will have been transformed. You will, I hope, be in the place I have arrived at and alive to the fact that working with as much dedication as the biochemists in the megalithic structures of the drug giants are the lesser known number of men and women, dedicating themselves, not to the cause of profit, but to exploration of the power of self healing, to deciphering the code of placebo and self imposed wellness.

Very fine scientists are working to disempower the myths those with vested interest impose upon us. I introduce you to the work of the modern day prophets, the most eloquent of the voices in placebo science and self help who teach us healing and well ness is much more complicated than surgery and pills.

I am not an academic and this is not intended to be an academic work. I have had to hang on by my shirt tails to some of the scientific results being written up at present, but reading the medical papers which document the results of the placebo medical experiments has undoubtedly been good for me. The findings of the placebo scientists allow me to see the potential I have as a human being to intervene in my own health. I believe the results from this area of science should be widely publicised. Indeed the results of the latest placebo experiments should be made required reading for everyone and anyone afflicted by illness and disease because the results would be inspiring to anyone who is ill.

How depleted in power and strength must anyone diagnosed with purportedly intractable disease feel? The test results obtained in a huge number of experiments dedicated to unravelling the secrets of the response within the body known as the 'placebo effect', do not provide health solutions. In many respects they complicate matters further because they document the inexplicable, but they do provide one thing; HOPE.

The power of the body to react to a useless sugar pill and effectively heal itself, illuminates, if, at present, only with a thin flickering light, the self healing power the body possesses. Much more work is needed to unlock the full secret of longevity and perpetual health for every human being but the results of this ongoing body of work are empowering and uplifting. The test results obtained in placebo trial experiments demonstrate the complexity of the body we possess, demonstrating that the true explanation of what 'cures' and restores a body to full health is still, to a large extent, beyond the grasp of modern science. Placebo trial results demonstrated to me the potential the body had for recalibration to 'healthy' if the mind was engaged in precisely the right way.

It was this corrective potential of the body my Ritual sought to harness. I can now see, several years down the line, that modern day healthcare with its emphasis on drug prescription and invasive medical techniques prevents us all from understanding the connection we could make with our own self if we tried.

Because of the manner in which modern healthcare is packaged delivered and processed we have lost touch with our primal instinct about what we need to keep us well. We have surrendered our power over our body to others and we have imposed an entire set of damaging beliefs upon ourselves our ancestors were never threatened by.

The focus of western medicine has shifted from any thought of self- healing, self- maintenance, self- restoration to outside intervention, to prescribing the latest drug or subjecting the body to the latest surgical technique. To techniques and practices that did not exist even twenty years ago and which will be outmoded and in many respects discredited in another twenty or less years as drugs come and go with patents expiring and the power to profit, from what is, the now accepted 'cure', reduced!

I would like protection for you and I from the pill makers and drug pedallers indifferent to the side effects their chemicals cause. I do not want you or I to suffer neediness and increasing dependence on drugs and the companies manufacturing them.

I want to be safe from those who do not know or understand the man I am. What it is that makes me tick, what my liver needs or my bile duct or any of my individual cells which may resemble those of a billion other beings but which are in fact only mine, sustained by me and which have my own particular individual way of operating and surviving and multiplying. My method which is mine and only mine because until genetic engineering perfects cloning and clones me there is indeed on the whole of this earth only one and only me and I would like that to be acknowledged and have a hand in my healing. Is that unreasonable? Is anyone out there in the corridors of healing as interested in my healing as I am?

I think not and that is why my Ritual once born was nurtured in to the effective tailored therapy it is today.

The Ritual has optimised my health, my wellbeing, my potential to enjoy my future. I am not aware of any evidence, drug company trial or government dictat that prohibits that or prevents me from saying to every one who is willing to give the Ritual a go, it really can change your life, health and energy levels for the better. Indeed I would go so far as to say the purchase of this book is one of the best investments you have ever made in your entire lifetime.

—————————— CHAPTER ONE ——————————

THE IMPORTANCE OF BELIEF

BELIEF

What is so important about belief?

Belief makes things work!

Think about your own life; the things that you have achieved. Not one thing you have ever been proud of, overjoyed by, or plain relieved to have behind you, would ever have been possible without the belief held in your subconscious mind that the intended objective was yours to deliver.

YOU BELIEVED YOU COULD DO IT AND SO YOU DID.

We are all born with the gift of belief within us.

Why is that?

Why is it if we put our mind to it we can believe in almost anything?

And why is it as soon as belief is engaged, the thing we believe in is ours?

You disagree?

The proviso is this, we must whole- heartedly, 100%, entirely, without doubt reserved, believe in the outcome we seek, and if we do, belief delivers it.

You disagree more vehemently!

Life is not that easy. You just cannot sit around believing in things and expect them to be delivered. If that worked you would win the lottery every Saturday night, live in a mansion, own a yacht!

I can imagine every one reading this book uttering these protestations to themselves, and my answer is this.

You do not win the lottery every Saturday night because you do not believe you will win. Belief is not engaged. In your mind there may be a hope of winning, but there is also an enormous quantity of doubt, and indeed disbelief that such a thing could occur.

Do most of us really believe we can own a yacht, or live in a mansion in Hollywood? Of course we don't. We don't believe in these things and so we remain on dry land, in a home the biggest mortgage we can secure, acquires for us.

Whose fault is that?

It is certainly not the fault of belief!

Belief is under used, left dormant in most minds, in most situations. What I ask you to do in performing the Ritual is to trigger it. Let it go; as you apply your self to the Ritual release the power of your belief and watch the results unfold.

Trust me, belief has built within it a force that confounds even the most brilliant minds in modern science, and the joyous thing is, we all possess it.

There must be a reason, don't you agree, that we are made in this way?

We are strings and chains of atoms, neurons and molecules. We are vibrant shapes intermingling and dancing on scans, vast seas of chemicals and yet we are inert, without action, plan or objective until we trigger belief. Belief is our driver. Think of that when I stress my Ritual cannot deliver one benefit to your life if you do not believe in it.

EVERYONE READING THIS BOOK IS GOING TO TAKE ON AGEING AND WIN.

Do you believe that?

If you don't perhaps it is time to remind yourself of what Henry Ford said:

'There is no man living that cannot do more than he thinks he can'.

The Ritual, that I am going to tell you about will work to impact beneficially on every aspect of your life; IF YOU BELIEVE IN IT.

Belief in the Ritual is the necessary detonator of a chain reaction of consequences that will change your life, health and prospects forever.

I can state this as a fact but I cannot begin to tell you why.

I have no idea why the consequences of believing are so dramatic, and why it is that a failure to believe results in uncertainty paralysis and apathy?

Scientists, academics and biologists are equally lost to explain the impact of belief.

Belief is subtle. It is buried within our awareness so that we forget about it. We do not even consider as we stand up from a chair and walk across the room our body believes it can do this. It can move. It can unfold the whole of the spine, push from the pelvis, take weight on the bones of the legs and feet and project itself wherever the mind directs it to. We take movement for granted and yet prior to performance of our every movement, our brain engages and we viscerally believe in the depths of our being, we are going to move.

Belief is the foundation we need if anything is to be achieved and what is more, the more intense our belief in an outcome, the greater the scale of our possible achievement.

BELIEF DELIVERS MIRACLES

English teenage ballet star Jack Widdowson who was attacked on an English street in 2011 knows this as does a young man from California Janne Kouri, the victim of an accident in the ocean in California in 2006. Both men suffered devastating injuries to the neck and spinal cord. Both independently made news headlines around the globe when their individual stunning recoveries, from what should, in both cases, have been a lifetime of paralysis, defied all medical prediction.

The two men had little in common save for the gravity of their initial injuries and their unwavering belief in their own recovery. Both Jack and Janne were told paralysis was the only expected consequence of the injuries they had suffered. Neither man was prepared to accept that fact. Two young men on either sides of the globe set apart from dozens of tragic others by a belief they held in their mind. They believed they would walk again and against all odds they both did.

There have been many reports of these cases. The one thing all the newspaper and internet accounts of the struggle of each man to recover make plain is that the faith of both Jack Widdowson and Janne Kouri in their own recovery was unshakeable. They believed, in the face of the grimmest medical predictions, they would recover, and they did.

What is our individual battle against ageing compared with the battle faced by these two young men?

Nothing!

I absolutely agree, and yet to many, beginning retirement, the onset of age, increasing infirmity, worsening aches and pain, the terror of memory loss, is everything.

It is a battle we each have to engage with and attitude, will and most importantly belief are the weapons we need if the battle is to be won. Belief in our own power to live differently, belief in the Ritual this book explains, is the key to positive change.

The secret is to believe.

Can you do that?

RELIGION

We really can believe in anything we choose.

Belief is in our gift. It is an innate ability we all possess.

Billions of people on this planet believe in a deity they have never seen, have little evidence for and whose teachings and principles they wish their individual lives to be governed by. Religions are diverse but all have one thing in common, complete and absolute faith. Many religions demand their followers to believe in a never witnessed, never personally experienced, being, the will and teachings of whom govern absolutely and determine rigorously, the boundaries of an entire lifetime. To the non- believer religious faith is incomprehensible. How can life be ruled, decisions made, actions governed, by facts that cannot be tested, challenged or truly ascertained?

The answer is faith. Determined and unquestioning belief in a greater being, idol, ideology or scheme that is able to save or curse the believer.

To believe in this way is to engage the brain in a particular way, and such faith brings results.

Belief brings peace, contentment, family structure, cohesion, shared worship. Belief holds communities and countries together just as opposing beliefs rip lives and countries apart.

To me religion demonstrates the awesome consequences of holding a belief with such certainty and conviction all doubt is excluded. It also demonstrates the ability of the human brain to form an unshakeable belief based on the most limited of information.

Religious belief is so deeply embedded within reason and consciousness it becomes the most powerful determinant of action, overriding even morality, contrary philosophy, and education. Outcomes are determined by information fed in to the ever -receptive brain. We are built to believe. We are built to react to what we believe in.

THE WHITE COATED SHAMAN

Shaman's still exist and have existed for centuries. There are today practising shamans in South America, Siberia, Mongolia, Korea, Japan and many parts of Central Asia. The Inuit peoples still use shamanism, and in many parts of Eastern Europe you can receive treatment from a shaman. Shamans are considered to be healers, medical men. Their method is to heal by healing the soul.

To heal a soul the shaman persuades the patient in front of him the remedy needed will come from the spirit world. The shaman acts as intermediary, communicating with spirits through ritual to obtain a cure. Dance, chant, burning herbs, and drumming are used, before the given diagnosis, that can cure or lead to death is delivered. The outcome in shamanism depends upon the news the shaman receives and communicates.

Pronouncements of malevolence in the patient, of disease invading the body, of a soul cursed, are delivered as news of terminal illness that can only lead to death.

Inevitably the cursed patient dies, believing the shaman's words.

Testimonies from shamanism provide evidence of the shaman delivering an end of life sentence to the patient together with exhortations to others in the community to change the way that they live if their own soul is to be saved. Stories abound of the shaman gathering new patients desperate not to be ill and the shaman's power strengthening with every diagnosis made. Right or wrong, healing or condemning, the shaman wins either way.

How many patients that die as a result of a shaman's words are really sick?

What effect do the words of the shaman have? Is all apocryphal, mere myth or is it true as the anthropologists say, that the diagnosis of a shaman, if negative, was the powerful influence on the mind of the man or woman treated that led to death.

We will never really know and in any event what has this quackery, this mysticism, to do with us? A patient cursed by news of a diseased soul. The shaman delivering the curse, the bad news that a soul will not be healed but go instead to hell. The quaintness, the devilry, the other worldliness, may seem ridiculous to us. How could these prophecies be accepted? Preposterous I hear you say; what relevance has this, in our time, in this 21st century world we are living in?

I understand your scepticism, but consider the shamans power, the position they held in individual societies, the magic of their spells, their books, their herbs, their insights in to the body and the mind of the person in front of them. They were the revered 'medical men'. The one's to have studied the body and the mind and to have found a way to heal it.

Sound familiar?

Consider a doctor today. Consider the ritual of examination, the pronouncements made, the diagnosis given as if a fact with all speculation and doubt concealed. The diagnosis accepted as the truth by the quivering patient, because it comes from a doctor in a white coat, with a stethoscope in place; the medical profession's ritualistic symbols of verification of everything that has been said. Consider the curse of the physician's terminal diagnosis, the impact of the language used.

'Three months to live'. 'I might give you a year'. 'You will not recover from this.'

Words handed out by the medical profession who principally are guessing. Imposing upon the very individual man or woman average survival rates, average outcomes. Hedging their bets, cautious not to deliver the very best to be hoped for. Instead pronouncing the worst. If one patient has survived post prostate cancer surgery for ten years but another has survived for two and the average time for survival is five and half years, what is it the patient will hear?

'I would give you two years', the inevitable words, the worst case scenario handed out by a doctor terrified of being sued. Doctors in the grip of lawyers and patients in the grip of the medical men.

Patients of the shaman and patients of a national health service, convinced, persuaded, believing, and belief the determinant of individual fate.

If you do not know already I hope by the time you finish this book you will understand, the body responds to the brain believing what it hears. Life that may have been lived can be taken by the power of belief. Imagine if the truth were always given? A patient told with optimism that the best that could be expected was ten years. Would the body give up at two?

Prognosis matters. Research has shown the manner in which a doctor delivers a prognosis to a patient matters. Doctors today really can be seen as white coated shamans. Every man or women held in thrall of the shaman or doctor's words is vulnerable to belief's power to determine outcome.

As in the ancient world the mother, child, father, accepted the shaman's words, the majority of us receive in exactly the same way a doctor's advice. We believe in exactly the same way. Is it not then a wonder that we die in exactly the same way.

Our minds are vulnerable to the information fed in to them. Negative information can have a dramatic effect but the good news is positive information is an even greater contender to produce even more dramatic results.

In Peru the Ayahuasqueros engage in the ritual use of 'ayahuasca', a psychedelic tea, which has been documented to cure everything from addiction to depression. Do you really think the tea contains every chemical compound known to man, laid down in complex formulae, in a pattern that can eradicate and heal every physical and psychological ill, or do you think it is the belief the Ayahuasqueros have in their tea that heals?

Is it not obvious?

THE POWER IS IN THE BELIEF.

THE HEALER AS CATALYST

I like this concept. I first came across it when reading a report by Ellen Warner MD of a conference held in Hamilton Canada in 1983.(1) This inter-disciplinary conference was intended to explore the

'Role of Belief in the Healing Process.' Conference delegates were theologians, physicians, psychiatrists, they collectively considered what evidence existed that faith/belief was effective in healing. Those attending the conference were all interested in determining how one makes a patient well. All were interested to explore if there should be an acknowledged role for faith/belief in the healing process; it being proposed by those from varying disciplines that an act of healing involves more than the use of scientific knowledge and technology to cure diseases. One shared contention explored by participants was that modern technologic medicine may occasionally cure disease but will never heal the ill patient.

Dr Joel Elkes defined 'wellness' as a state of 'connectedness' or 'wholeness'. He believed when healing occurs, 'the healer serves as a catalyst that connects the patient to his own resources'.

I find the approach of Dr Elkes inspiring. Not only was he a mainstream physician, (a psychiatrist and philospher,) prepared to examine conventional medicine, to see if it or some other factor was the key to health and healing, he was also willing to identify a role for the patient and the patient's own belief system in the healing process. Dr Elkes, thirty two years ago, recognised the power a patient had over his or her belief, over his or her 'wellness'. He recognised the power of the mind, and the belief held within it, not just the chemical reaction of the pill or the neatness of the surgeons scalpel in delivering what it takes to be well.

WHAT DO WE BELIEVE ABOUT AGEING?

What do we believe about our human lifespan?

About how we will age and the control we will have over our life as our decline becomes evident?

Does not science, medicine, society and our every bred instinct create the conscious expectation that from the moment of mid life, we will inexorably decay, decrease in strength, ability and value, contribute less to others and progress powerlessly towards the end point of our life, our death?

Isn't that how we believe things will be? And do we not also consider that we are helpless to control the state we will be in when we progress to such an ending?

It is the truth isn't it? You believe it, I believe it, it is what we are educated to expect.

But it is not necessarily true. It can be otherwise and the sooner you adjust those, in the main conditioned and outdated patterns of thought, to promote a new position, the sooner your life will change.

We can be magnificent at 103. Believe that if you need something to believe in.

What powerlessness do we imbue our self with when we believe during our every conscious moment we have no control over the inevitable frailties of age?

Persuading ourselves we are doomed to finish our existence at some unknown but certain point to be determined by our physical collapse is bad for our health. How can such a negative pattern of belief co-exist with an extension of our lifetime or maintenance of our vigour and youthfulness?

If we are to live for a long time in good health we have to change our thoughts.

As you age, be elated. A society that shuns the aged has it wrong. Societies in which the aged are revered have it right. Celebrate your wisdom, your accumulated life experience, the development of your spirit and feel content.

Re-shape your thinking. Deliver new messages to your consciousness.

No longer consider

AGE MEANS INFIRMITY

RETIREMENT IS FOR SLOWING DOWN

I WILL ONE DAY BE UNABLE TO CARE FOR MYSELF

OLD AGE IS FOR INACTIVITY AND DORMANCY

This is limited thinking and if you want to benefit from the Ritual you have to discover thinking that is unlimited.

LIFE WITHOUT LIMITS

In some parts of this world the abhorrent practice of enslaving human beings still exists. I cannot imagine a society that tolerates a human being chained, obliged to work at the dictate of others, but with equal abhorrence I cannot tolerate free human beings capable of independent thought and action enslaving themselves with their thoughts.

So many people in their sixties and seventies revel in being old. They create age for themselves as if it is a coat that will protect them.

'I am not as fit as I used to be'

'I do what I can'

'It's a bad day today, I've got that pain I get in my back'

I hear these comments in the supermarket, in the queue at the bank, from men and women who are patently physically younger than myself but who are locking themselves up in a self built prison of age, laying the foundations and the bricks, thought by negative thought.

It is 2014, many of us who are now sixty will live to 2054. Get the hang of it.

2054 is a long way away, if you want to enjoy every day between now and then, begin now, think differently.

Thoughts about the onset of decrepitude at fifty or sixty or even seventy five are not helpful they are literally going to break your back and render you infirm a long time before you need to be.

IT IS NECESSARY TO CHANGE YOUR MINDSET

If you are prepared to follow the Ritual I describe your mindset will change. It will be the first thing to alter and this alteration of mindset will change the rest of your life.

Grasp that and youth is yours. Wellness will be yours. It is your choice.

Imagine the consequence for your body of removing the limits upon your expectations as to the health and vitality you will possess at 90, 100, 105.

Imagine the jubilance of the body if all that were fed in to the mind was the message that there is no certain end date? No need for physical decline, in fact the converse, the possibility of physical improvement and rejuvenation?

Most of us believe we can achieve certain things but not others. We believe we can attain a certain standard of health and fitness for a certain time but not forever. Most, certainly the majority of us, believe that some how the health that we possess is not our own responsibility. It is as if we consider the situation is out of our hands, governable by external factors and even worse by remote ungovernable fate

IT IS NOT TRUE!

We can intervene.

All it takes is an altered set of beliefs.

The majority of us do not believe as young men and women that we can walk on hot coals or dive from the highest ridge nature ever created. Some can, but not us! Isn't that what is instilled in the centre of a mind, when the mind and the subconscious cosy up to have a chat? We are limited. We as a human being can do certain things but not others. Only birds can fly.

LIMITS LIMITS LIMITS

But what of the child trained to believe in the unlimited nature of their being? The yogi child, brought up to walk on coals, the child of the amazon, brought up to dive from the ridge. These human beings have the same physiology, same organs and brain and tissues as us but they have a different perspective. Such children defy any concept of human limitation. Limits for them are overriden by belief, by affirmation and confirmation from the adults around them that hot coals are nothing to fear, that the highest rock shelf on the mountain is a step only towards a goal that can be attained.

These children are taught to believe in their ability to walk across burning coals without the coal having the power to burn them. They are taught to believe in the capability of almost flight to land and penetrate water as if they are a cormorant, never once considering the leap, the impact with the water may injure them. The prospect of injury does not enter their mind. Their mind has no room for it, it is too busy believing in technique and successful outcome. To such children coals are not something that can damage them. The ridge is not a shelf so high that death could occur on impact if only one centimetre of their neck were out of line. They do not see danger because they do not believe in anything other than their own ability to do the thing required. The mind is brainwashed by belief and the outcome is achieved.

These otherwise physiologically identical human beings defy conventional human limits. They are trained to feats beyond the reach of other humans who have the same physical and mental structures available within them, not simply because they are courageous or because of unique physical athleticism, but because they convince their mind.

THEY BELIEVE THEY CAN WALK ON HOT COALS

THEY BELIEVE THEY CAN DIVE LIKE A CORMORANT FROM A LEDGE

AND THEY CAN !!

The only difference between you and they is the belief they hold in their mind. It is this that I want you to understand before you begin your journey with me to comprehend the Ritual that I have created.

If you want the Ritual to work

BELIEVE YOU ARE AGELESS

BELIEVE EVERY ADDITIONAL YEAR OF YOUR LIFE WILL BE ENRICHING

BELIEVE YOU ARE IN CONTROL OF THE HEALTH THAT YOU POSSESS

And you will be, and what is even more exciting, the limits you have previously placed upon your own life, will simply fall away.

It is necessary as you perform my Ritual to remember only one thing. Human limitation is not set within a human blue print, it is propaganda etched inside a head. Inside a mind.

ANOTHER WAY

En masse we believe we are born to age and decay, but what if we are wrong?

All of us!

What if we, the bunch of credible individuals that we are, with our belief in ageing and decay are quite simply wrong? And what if the error is bigger than that? What if the scientists, biologists and academics who teach us that we have no control over our health or degeneration, are also wrong. What if science really does not know, or what if science knows something but not enough and there are in fact unlimited variables, endless possibilities, for every human being to defy the *en masse* expectation?

John Robbins, in his masterpiece, *Healthy at 100*, documents the lives of peoples who do not fit the stereotypical matrix of expectations imposed upon the aged. (2) John Robbins tells us of the people of Abkhasia in the Caucasus, 'where people are healthier at ninety than most of us are at middle age'. Of the people of Vilacamba, in Ecuador, described by John Robbins as, 'The Valley of Eternal Youth', a place in which, ' heart disease and dementia do not exist'. In Hunza at the northernmost tip of Pakistan, people, ' dance in their nineties', and 'cancer, diabetes and asthma are unknown'. In the Japanese state of Okinawa, 'there are more centenarians than anywhere else in the world'.

John Robbins describes the diet and lifestyle of each of the peoples observed and endeavours to draw conclusions for the rest of mankind about what can be learned from these diverse peoples who defy any logical expectation of limitation upon longevity and health. I refer to John Robbin's work not only to ensure all readers are acquainted with it, (because even reading his books are good for the health), but to make the point that there is another way.

I want every one reading this book to believe that.

Old age does not have to be stultifying, depressing and bleak. We do not have to race towards decrepitude believing that is our lot. We have to believe in our longevity, and in the possibility of continuing wellness. We will all die, but we can die in good shape, quietly and at peace having been fully alive.

After years of performing my Ritual I know this to be the truth. We can all descend gracefully through an enriching later life and if it is our desire we can still be paragliding or mountain climbing or ball room dancing on the last day that we are alive.

The Ritual taps in to a life sustaining energy.

Prior to imposing the discipline of my daily Ritual upon myself I too felt I was running against the clock, ticking off the days until I died. I was a man mapped by my physical self, by the strengths or weaknesses of my biology. It was as if my brain was apart, helpless, an inactive observer of my decline.

If my brain engaged at all it was in a negative way. The beliefs my head delivered reminded me life would become more challenging as the years went by. I understood, because I told myself, time and time again, there would be a drying out of my skin, a hardening of my arteries, a slow atrophying of every organ I possessed. Regardless of what I felt about it, incapacity and senility would find me and reduce me until my death.

What credit did I give to the power of my belief to deliver a different message? What information was I feeding to my sub-conscious? The unconscious mind that in its ceaseless activity cannot be charted but is at all times dominant, controlling every action within my life.

What before invention of my Ritual did I make of the concept of my soul? The object without fixed position or clear explanation that adds to every life experience, something intangible, frequently illuminating, always questioning, voicing from within every human being, something beyond thought, that is neither emotion, or hard neurological response, but something in between. Something ephemeral which connects us to an energy beyond our own life. An energy that I can only comprehend as the energy of the unending Universe; that is all, from matter to non matter, from darkness to light.

Something inexplicable is contained within each and every one of us that science has never managed to reduce to an explicable biological system. That is the magnificent fact. That is the reason the Ritual had to be written because every day I tap in to a power that has nothing at all to do with my physiology, my flesh and bloodness of being, but which is an overriding force available to each and every one of us, that has the power within it to change a life.

I am so overwhelmed by what I have discovered about my own innate power to slow down the ageing process, to improve my health, to alter my outlook on my future, enhance my comprehension of the errors and wrong turns and limiting beliefs of my past, that I have no choice but to tell the world about it and this book is my attempt to do just that.

CHAPTER TWO

THE PHENOMENON THAT IS THE PLACEBO EFFECT

WHAT EXACTLY IS A PLACEBO?

I knew vaguely. I understood it was to do with a patient getting better even when they had not been given a real pill. I believed that it was something to do with illness being all in the mind. That is what I thought. The limits of my knowledge, before I felt my Ritual having a dramatic effect on my health and well being and I decided to investigate, what is, the phenomenon of placebo further.

What I have found out about the emerging science of placebo and the placebo response astounds me and makes me question the basis of mainstream western medicine and also induces in me a type of alarm that the multi billions dedicated to keeping a national health service upright are not in part dedicated to investigating further the ability of the body to self heal. Well that is not self heal, entirely, without help, but to heal with the direction and intervention of the mind.

We can heal ourselves. In part, placebo trials and investigative placebo science, demonstrate this. We have within us a mechanism that can be triggered for self- healing but even in this technologically rich decade of medical investigation and billion dollar funded research no one knows the precise nature of this mechanism or the relevant trigger to activate the physiological systems within us to make the process begin.

I cannot claim that I have solved the grand mystery of self healing but I do believe my Ritual works in the same way placebos do. I believe the same healing mechanism is engaged by sugar pills and by my Ritual exercises. I believe through the conditioning power of my Ritual I provoke my body to repair and maintain itself and even cure itself of ills just as ineffective starch and sugar pill substitutes cure pain and impact upon disease.

I genuinely believe we can make ourselves ill and vulnerable to disease and conversely we can boost our immune system and keep ourselves well; third party forces, such as accident, devastating injury, terrorist attack, rail crash, and other traumatic events beyond our control, aside.

Placebo trials show that human beings can respond as effectively to sugar pills, to sham surgery, to inert tablets, as they can to complex pharmaceutical concoctions. Not only can the human body and mind compete with pharmaceuticals it can out do the pharmaceutical under trial to such an extent that the tablet or pill in production never comes to market because it cannot be demonstrated that the clinical impact of the pill or tablet a drug company proposes is better than the response of the human body and mind to nothing, to simply the suggestion, belief and expectation, that a pill or treatment has been given or surgery performed that will fix things.

DID YOU KNOW THAT?

Have you read in the newspapers about the gift that is yours, that I firmly believe can extend your life, maintain the health of your body, slow down, to the extent of near defeat the ageing process? Have you seen alongside the dual carriageways in the centre of your town, beside the hospital blocks, the huge edifices dedicated to understanding the science of self healing, to triggering a placebo response?

Of course you haven't. What devastation would occur if science were made to work on the secret of self healing? If research projects were committed to persuading the average man or woman in the street the secret to their future health and longevity lay within them?

What scale of recession would occur if we did not need the NHS; or not the NHS as it is today, but a reduced size institution with billions cut from its budget, existing to provide care only in the event of traumatic or colossal injury?

That is, in the event of our bodies being assaulted by agents, third parties or events inevitably beyond our control.

According to the NHS Choices website only Walmart, the Chinese Peoples' Liberation Army and the Indian Railway have more employees than the British NHS. Not allowing for the tens of thousands feeding the system from their employment in pharmaceuticals. What if the technique of self- healing could be learned and implemented, what then of the structure of our country? The multi billions invested in NHS structures and pharmaceutical stocks and shares?

We are so heavily invested in ill health; the structure of our job market and society is so dependent upon illness, we can't just wipe illness out.

Or can we?

Well I believe we can dramatically engage with the shape that we are in, with the thoughts that we carry, and the environment that we create within ourselves. It is clear to me the manner in which we engage with our own self, body and mind and soul, has an impact upon the wellness we possess and the length and quality of our lives.

I believe that the results of placebo trials conducted globally should be widely publicised and included in every school curriculum. Self -healing should not be some notion of eccentrics, sidelined and derided, it should be honoured and taught and investigated and pursued.

Of course it is in many disciplines in the East but when there is an effort to transport self healing techniques to the West and to incorporate them into day to day Western mainstream medicine and living the practitioners concerned are labelled, 'alternative', 'charlatans', 'quacks'. Try raising self -healing with your GP on your next visit, or slip it in to a consultation with a hospital consultant to see what response you will receive. It is as if there is a wall between mainstream medical responses and the possibility of healing based on mind body connection that is greater and more substantial, more tirelessly constructed, than the wall that stood in Berlin or the wall that remains, extending across China.

I believe opinions must change; those who believe in self healing are not invaders with opinions that will decimate the culture that stands in tact behind the wall of chemical and technological medicine, they are insightful and gifted beings who are ahead, curious, and inspired, by the responses they have seen in the body when the mind is stimulated in a particular way. Those studying and writing about the ability of the human body to heal itself are not in fact magicians or charlatans but magi carrying in knowledge which should be received, built upon and cherished.

21

I want to briefly look at what is being achieved in this world of scientific experiment. I do not collate all of the scientific results available. It is not necessary, many books are on the market today which deal in depth with placebo research, providing a full and scientifically analytical description of on going work. This book is not about the placebo effect. I want to introduce my readers to what is happening in placebo science as a precursor to explaining how my Ritual works, quite simply because the benefits my Ritual delivers are more likely to be accepted by those already familiar with the extraordinary demonstration of human potential sugar pills provide us with.

The test results I acquaint you with should in my opinion be labelled ASTOUNDING HEALTH GIVING NEWS and made available in bound pamphlets at the entrance to every ward in every hospital of every state health provider to provide hope to those who lie in the beds within.

PLACEBO: THE WORK OF UNDERSTANDING

Socrates and Plato thought about and discussed the placebo response. Hundreds of years before the birth of Christ, two Greek philosophers, student and pupil, announced the response was real.

'*The cure for a headache was a kind of leaf, which required to be accompanied by a charm, and if a person would repeat the charm at the same time as he used the cure, he would be made whole; but that without the charm the leaf would be of no avail.*'

Socrates according to Plato from Dialogues of Plato.

I find it almost wondrous that several centuries before the birth of Christ, individuals living on this Earth were discussing the potency of a cure when the cure in question was linked to a Ritual, to the manner in which the cure was delivered.

All that time ago it was known there was more to the workings of the body and to medicine than the straightforward imbibing of a medicine. What truly astonishes me, is that in the millennia that have passed since Plato and Socrates discussed the matter, unravelling why medicines work more effectively, if wrapped up in a ritual or a spell, has been a priority for a miniscule percentage of the scientific and medical profession.

Most are interested in perfecting new drug cocktails, in profit. It is the minority of those involved with science and medicine that care about the charm and the ritual and the spell. It is a matter worth celebrating that in our time the voice of this minority is getting louder and louder and the results of their practical experiments becoming harder and harder to deny.

What makes us heal? Scientists and physicians know it is not just the drugs or the event of surgery. They may not tell us, the populace, the uninformed, but the complexity of how to heal, as opposed to treat, is analysed and set down in bound volumes of medical experiment and thousands of pages of clinical trial results.

We can heal ourselves.

Often, from all sorts of ills and every practising medic in the world knows that to be the case. It is even on the syllabus at medical school, bundled up, packaged and taught as the placebo effect.

What actually is the placebo effect?

Well in my trawl through the literature of placebo it has been variously described. It is 'a trinity of hope, expectation and belief'. It is something, which occurs 'independently of the intentions of health professionals'. It is 'a spontaneous improvement in health occurring in the absence of an active chemical.' It is 'a sugar pill, a sham surgical procedure, a fake therapy, producing real therapeutic benefits'.

It does, whichever way you look at it, appear to be something that is real. A tangible measurable response of the body to information received by the brain.

In 1955 a Harvard Professor of anaesthesia Henry K Beecher published *The Powerful Placebo*. It was Henry K Beecher's conclusion that:

'It is evident that placebos have a high degree of therapeutic effectiveness in treating subjective responses.....a real therapeutic effect being produced in 35.2% of cases'(1)

All those years ago Henry Beecher a respected physician was telling the world drugs cure, but in 35.2% of cases, for conditions, in which the patient's subjective assessment of how they feel is relevant, placebos cure also. 35.2% of patients given nothing at all feel better.

This conclusion was reached from Henry Beecher's work with 1000 patients over 15 studies covering a wide range of areas: wound pain, the pain of angina pectoris, headache, nausea, drug induced mood change, anxiety and tension, and the common cold.

There is anecdotal evidence that Henry Beecher became interested in the effects of placebo medicine while tending to injured troops under bombardment from the German army in WWII. Some accounts of Henry Beecher's service indicate that morphine supplies ran out during the course of the bombardment of a battalion of US soldiers and out of sympathy nurses tending the wounded administered saline substitutes to soldiers suffering massive wounds in place of morphine.

In some accounts it is written that Henry Beecher watched pain - ridden soldiers improve when only given saline injections. The soldiers believing they were being given morphine. I cannot say and we will probably never know if saline was administered in this way. It is at odds with Henry Beecher's own account in his writings in which he describes tending to soldiers with serious and grave wounds and being surprised that such soldiers did not request pain relief, their subjective appreciation of pain not correlating with the objective reality of the pain they should have been experiencing as a result of the wounds that they had suffered.

The power of morphine is in Beecher's terms, '*a placebo effect plus its drug effect': 75% of a group in severe post operative pain are satisfactorily relieved by a large dose of morphine, but 35% are relieved by placebo'.*

Beecher wrote that placebos are most effective when the stress of the illness, (anxiety suffered or pain suffered by the patient) is greatest. All of Beecher's work demonstrated placebos being their most effective when there is great significance for the patient in the drug that is given. In Beecher's terms the opinion a patient forms that a drug is the 'latest', 'most effective', 'most expensive', would have an effect on the healing the tablet delivers.

Henry Beecher's early assessment of the power of a placebo substitute has been shown, in later placebo trials, to be less than generous. On occasion, up to 72 % of patients receiving a placebo substitute, (that is a tablet containing nothing) instead of an active pharmaceutical have demonstrated an improvement in symptoms equal to those receiving the active drug being trialled. (2)

The triggering of a placebo response, as we shall see, is a hugely complex matter.

Scientists now know placebo responses vary depending on the characteristics of the individual selected for inclusion in a placebo control group. Responses vary across clinical trials and most surprisingly placebo effects vary within different countries and in the trialling of different diseases.

Amongst the many variables one thing is plain, the placebo response baffles medics, scientists, professors, and researchers. It has for over five decades created theories as to its workings but no real solution.

Daniel Moerman and Wayne Jonas in their paper, published in 2002, *Deconstructing the Placebo Effect and Finding the Meaning Response.(3),* refer to some of the academic effort put in to decoding placebo.

'*There is a renewed interest in placebos and the placebo effect- on their reality, their ethics, their place in medicine, or not, both in and out of the clinic and academy. The U.S National Institutes of Health recently sponsored a large conference called "Science of the Placebo". At least five serious books on the subject, plus a book of poetry, and a novel, each entitled The Placebo Effect – have been published since 1997. In the past ten years, the National Library of Medicine has annually listed an average of 3972 scholarly papers with the key words,"placebo", "placebos"or "placebo effect" with a low of 3362 papers in 1992 and a high of 4814 in 2000"*

It is clear to me scientists, professors, academics all want to unravel the placebo response. And it is clear another dozen years or so after Moerman & Jonas published their paper it is still not known what the placebo response is or how it is triggered. It is important when you consider the merits of my Ritual that you grasp that.

Why?

Because I have seen that my Ritual stimulates my mind to interact with my body to deliver therapeutic benefits just as effectively as a trick of medicine, through delivery of a sugar pill or a sham act of surgery, provokes the mind to stimulate the body to heal.

How my Ritual achieves this I do not know. I cannot begin to understand the bio mechanics, which does not mean I am stupid, it means I am alongside some of the best medical researchers in the world, because, as I write this, nobody knows.

My Ritual harnesses a number of powerful techniques any one of which has been shown to deliver therapeutic benefits. Through the combination of these known therapies and the systematic application of my Ritual to my body I have triggered in myself a rejuvenating self healing response which I believe is the same elusive bodily response witnessed in placebo trials when those who should not heal, because they have not been cured by pills or surgery, effectively heal themselves.

That is a huge statement. But I make it after years of performing my daily Ritual and observing within myself the benefits my Ritual has delivered.

According to any assessment society makes of me I should not be as flexible, lithe, vigorous, ambitious, alert, fit, (in cardiovascular and performance terms) as I am. I should not think as I do, move as I do, dress as I do, look as I do, live as I do. I am living as a man in his fifties but I am seventy years of age. I am disease free. I have no joint pain. My hair grows. My libido is intact. How can I explain these things to others? What do I do that others of the same age, but aged, are not doing?

It is my Ritual that sets me apart.

My Ritual orchestrates, directing my mind to intervene in my health, just as the mind of those in placebo trials is captured by the information fed in to it and stimulated to interact with the body that is ill. In both cases the consequences of provocation of the mind are unlikely, unpredictable and difficult to comprehend, but in both cases the outcome of the process is overwhelmingly beneficial.

In a sequel to this book I want to be able to explain why my Ritual works, describing the bio-mechanical processes stimulated that invigorate my biology and hold back ageing and disease.

I am not going to come up with an explanation on my own. I rely on those researching within this area of science to help me, to carry me with them, as their research brings breakthroughs, because I am one man alone and I can not solve this on my own.

The good news for my sequel is that decoding the power of placebos, and by analogy, of home spun rituals that preserve and invigorate, is a matter of importance to science. In 2002 a vast array of experts involved in placebo research prepared and presented papers now collated in a BMJ publication, *The Science of Placebo: Toward an Interdisciplinary Research Agenda.*

This work, in my humble, non academic opinion, provides any one of us, who is interested, with much of what is known today about placebos.

Anne Harrington, Professor of the History of Science at Harvard University, caused me to sit up and pay attention to her words as she brought home to me that a placebo response is not something only to be obtained from ingestion of sugar pills.

In explaining what may be relevant to an understanding of the placebo response, Anne Harrington instructs any scientist willing to listen; (4)

'We might want to pay some attention to what I call, "sightings": phenomena that do not generally get catalogued as examples of the placebo effect, but that we might all agree have, " something to do with it". " Sightings, in other words, are fauna that live in some larger territory of human psychobiological functioning where the placebo effect makes its home as well. By expanding our vision to make room for at least some near relations of that effect, we may find ourselves inspired to ask questions about that larger territory that otherwise might not have occurred to us.'

The "sightings", Anne Harrington refers to, which she considers may have some relevance to consideration of the placebo effect, and should therefore be taken into consideration when thought is given to what the placebo effect is, are amongst the most interesting facts I have come across in my quest to understand what is the multi faceted nature of the potential self healing capability within all of us.

Anne Harrington cites examples of hospital patients, given a hospital bed near to a window that looks on to a beautiful view, healing up to 7 – 9 weeks sooner than patients with identical medical conditions allocated a room with a window overlooking the hospital car park.

More poignantly she describes a number of Cambodian widows, living in the United States, having lost husbands or children to the massacre of the killing fields, suffering blindness, not due to any detectable pathology of the eye but because "they had cried until they could not see". They were blind from grief, not for an explicable optical reason.

Many "sightings", are listed but the final one I include here is that of the ability of a human being to postpone the timing of their death in order to celebrate a symbolically important religious festival, to attend an important family celebration or event, or to complete unfinished business.

It is not suggested death can be timed, blindness onset or healing spurred, by an intrinsic gift we have within us to self regulate how our body responds. The examples are given as examples of self inflicted healing and harm only but I suggest what each demonstrates is more profound and hopeful than something that simply widens the debate about placebo. I believe the 'sightings' listed take us to another place, and that place I consider is comfortably close to that in which I find myself when my Ritual does its work.

Anne Harrington's "sightings" provide anecdotal evidence of medically inexplicable acts of accelerated self-healing, self injury, or sustenance of cellular activity, which mainstream medicine cannot provide any straightforward mainstream medical answer for. That does not mean the described events did not happen and it does not mean the process triggered by the individuals concerned is not demonstrative of the gift within each and every human being to self heal or self harm. To regulate the human body in a compassionate homespun way rather than farming out the task to a megalithic state health provider.

It is the ability of the mind to engage with the task of bodily repair that is, in my opinion, key. What happens in my brain when I commit myself to perform my therapeutic Ritual defies explanation because the brain and the expression of our intelligence through the power of our mind is not fully understood. Indeed the mind delivers outcomes, that are, time and time again, in terms of human biology, inexplicable.

If we are to age, we should all age in the same way. Regardless of race, creed or geography we are all more or less made in the same way. No stunning differences in physiology or the biology of our cells, explain why outcomes are so dramatically different depending on the thoughts our brains contain and the mindset we each personally develop.

Let's consider the menopause; and the varying response of women from different cultures to its onset. In the West there is a borderline obsession with the repeated description of symptoms women can expect to suffer at any point from their late forties onwards. Women are told to expect devastating and embarrassing, 'hot flushes', 'night sweats', 'emotional instability', 'memory loss'. In other words to prepare for a crisis induced by changing hormonal levels. Women are fed the expectation of unavoidable and prolonged symptoms of hormonal chaos. The message from the medicinal world of the West is delivered against the backdrop of vigorous debate about the benefits and drawbacks to a woman of commencing a course of hormone replacement therapy, which may damage her cardio vascular system, impact upon her liver and raise her susceptibility to strokes and various cancers.

The obvious consequence of such broadcasting of gloom is that in our society very substantial numbers of women are plagued by just the symptoms they are told to expect. With any additional random symptomology experienced by a women over fifty set down at the feet of the menopause as agent and creator, regardless of the existence of any causal link between symptoms experienced and hormonal imbalance. In brief most western women are told to expect to suffer when they reach a certain age and by jove, in the western hemisphere, they do. In the East, by contrast, little is expected, little is noticed, and in the majority of women little is experienced.

Daniel Moerman a medical anthropologist from the University of Michigan in his paper *Deconstructing the Placebo Effect and Finding the Meaning Response* urges us to consider the placebo response as an individuals response to the meaning in the medicine that is given. Daniel Moerman reviews the areas within medicine in which the meaning attached to a particular treatment by a patient affects illness or healing. He presents the following example of mortality rates among Chinese Americans diagnosed with lymphatic cancer which I believe can be considered in similar terms to Anne Harrington's 'sightings', as providing insight in to what a placebo response actually is.

Daniel Moerman cites the case of Chinese Americans born in an 'earth' year, as defined by the Chinese calendar. Those born in an 'earth' year are recognised in China to have a higher risk of susceptibility to death occurring as a result of a lump, bump or tumour. Daniel Moerman points out that studies of Chinese Americans suffering from lymphatic cancer have shown the average age at death amongst those in the sample group born in an 'earth' year to be 59.7 years of age. By contrast Chinese Americans born in a year not categorised by the Chinese calendar as a year likely to expose them to just the illness they are suffering from, have an average life expectancy of 63.6 years.

That is when the mind has not been affected by a belief in susceptibility to death from a disease, such as the very one that has been diagnosed, almost four years further life, albeit in the same diseased state, can be anticipated.

Moerman gives the following explanation:

' *No such differences were evident in a large series of "whites" who died of similar causes in the same period. The intensity of the effect was shown to be correlated with "the strength of commitment to traditional Chinese culture." These differences in longevity (up to 6% or 7% difference in the length of life!) are not due to having Chinese genes, but to having Chinese ideas, to knowing the world in Chinese ways.*'

Anne Harrington concludes her listing of " sightings", by stating:

'*....the point by now should be clear. There is an old Chinese saying that speaks of a finger pointing to the moon and then exhorts us to avoid a common human error by confusing the pointer with the target: "Look at the moon, not the finger that points." What we begin to learn when we engage with our historical legacies is that sugar pills are not themselves the point: they are instead themselves pointers to an arena of human functioning bigger than themselves.*'

It inspires me to know that a woman so greatly respected for her work as a scientist is prepared to say that the placebo response is evidence of some greater mechanism at work within every being. I ask you to remember her words when you endeavour, in the performance of your daily Ritual, to access the potential within yourself.

If you remain sceptical of the benefits my Ritual delivers, if at this stage in your life and at this point in this book, the thesis I propose is still an unlikely proposition, I ask you to return to the neurologically and biologically tested proposition that a human being uses only 10% of the capacity within their brain to sustain the type of life we are all known to live.

This is a tested fact, and if this has indeed been established is it not likely we possess within ourselves a power we do not yet recognise or fully understand? A power which we can, I believe, only come to understand and utilise, by focusing upon it, and endeavouring, if only in an amateur way, to access and apply it, each and every day that we live.

THE PLACEBO RESPONSE OBSERVED

One thing to understand about placebos is that before they were even talked about or scientifically researched, they existed. The placebo response was not invented in pharmaceutical drug trials or by Henry Beecher in 1955; placebos have been with us since the beginning of mankind. Their unacknowledged potential was probably healing cavemen or bronze age hunters of back pain!

It is only in the last handful of decades that we have had chemically potent drugs such as antibiotics able to fight bacteria and infection and to leave real traces of their workings in every bodily system. Prior to the 1950's few pharmacologically complex drugs existed. Most drugs dispensed would not now be given, their curative potential being dubious, but they were given in earlier decades, and gladly received, because they were all that was around. And they produced both cures and results. They cannot have done it through powerful medical efficacy, they did it, these old fashioned useless drugs, because of the potential they all had to trigger a placebo response.

Antibiotics are today given reluctantly by GP's at the insistence of patients to deal with viruses, and any unexplained symptomology that cannot be shifted by other means. They are even administered to cure the common cold. Antibiotics cannot do this, they cannot have any effect upon the cold virus or influenza or many conditions a patient presents with but every patient greatfully receives the antibiotic given and amazingly within hours of taking it, for absolutely no clinical reason, begins to feel well.

Patients believe, because the pill they have in their hand is an antibiotic, (that tablet that can only be obtained by production of a signed prescription, by delivery of this document to a pharmacist who unlocks a cabinet to put a pill in a patient's hand) that an effective remedy has been delivered.

The charm is woven, a pill that is not designed to have any pharmacological impact on a virus, dissipates its potency, the lack lustre unwellness that has beset a patient for weeks, that cannot have been touched by the antibiotic, is gone and the patient is made well.

A magician may as well have waved a wand. The same process is engaged, the mysterious process of self healing triggered, that has to do with the arrival of the patient's mind in the treatment room, and nothing at all to do with the antibiotic pill.

You will begin to understand the placebo effect is a phenomenon worthy of study. The consequences for mankind for understanding what triggers a body to heal itself is worth not only billions and billions of pounds in terms of savings on healthcare, it is the key to ending scarcity, health lotteries, and inadequate access to health care in emerging countries. Placebo; the remedy that would change every life on this planet and yet it is only in the last fifteen years of so, as a result of the work of a handful of scientists, (who in my opinion everyone alive should honour as the good guys,) that the placebo response has been studied for its own sake.

The Harvard Magazine- February 2013 Edition, makes the point:

'For the last 15 years, Kaptchuk and fellow researchers have been dissecting placebo interventions – treatments that, prior to the 1990's, had been studied largely as foils to "real" drugs. To prove a medicine is effective, pharmaceutical companies must show not only that their drug has the desired effects, but that the effects are significantly greater than those of a placebo control group. Both groups often show healing results, Kaptchuk explains, yet for years, " We were struggling to increase drug effects while no one was trying to increase the placebo effect".

Ted Kaptchuk at Harvard University is in my opinion one of the best of the good guys. In 2012 Ted Kaptchuk and his colleagues from Harvard University created the Program in Placebo Studies, run by the Beth Israel Deaconess Medical Centre. This is presently the only multi- disciplinary institute dedicated solely to placebo study.

It astounds me that research work to understand placebo is more or less in its infancy. For decades untold wealth has been dedicated to the production of effective pills and potions but no one until almost the turn of this century has asked why the body is able to heal itself.

Due to the entire focus of modern medicine resting upon the belief that the body is an entity to be repaired from without, through the imbibing of liquids or the swallowing of pills, or the passive acceptance of radiotherapy, chemotherapy, or newly developed surgical procedures, we have shifted our focus away from our interior being to external cure.

My Ritual, when it was first created, was my attempt to shift my perspective back, to where it is now, to where, after several years of performing my Ritual, I am even more persuaded, it properly should be, upon my interior self.

I believe to begin to decode the placebo response we need to look within. All we need is within us. These words have become my mantra. I believe they add something to the ongoing scientific debate about what placebo is, how it is triggered and the bio chemical response generated that allows the body to present differently, to present as if it is cured and well.

IT IS NOT ALL ABOUT SUGAR PILLS

A part of my Ritual is dedicated to persuading and convincing my mind of a certain outcome I expect to achieve. My Ritual involves the delivery of messages through affirmation, to that part of my consciousness I hope to engage in healing work. I condition myself to expect a certain outcome. Auto-conditioning may be scientifically challenging to the medical community. I cannot comment upon that but I can state it is what I do. I shape my message and I deliver it. Placebo experiments have shown me that the messages patients receive from physicians matter and I calculate it is the same with my Ritual. I want to be well not ill, happy, not depressed. My message delivered by affirmation expresses the conclusion I want to achieve, and just as the nature of a message a patient receives changes medical results I believe the overwhelming optimism of the message I deliver to myself keeps me in good health and good shape.

The pain a patient experiences can be affected by the message delivered by a physician as to the likely affect of the pain killer the patient has been given. A strong message which asserts definite pain relief will occur will result in a patient experiencing less pain as compared to the pain reduction observed if a weak equivocal message is delivered by a physician which suggests *perhaps* there will be some pain relief.

This holds true even if both patient groups, that is patient group and control group, are given an inert sugar pill. The group receiving a sugar pill, the strength of which to deal with pain, is enforced at the time of its delivery to the patient, experience pain relief, whereas those given sugar and a weak message as to the possible but not definite potential of the tablet to relieve their pain continue to suffer. The placebo trial in question going a long way to establishing it is the message a clinician delivers that provides the pathway to recovery, and not the pill.

A positive consultation with a patient as opposed to a negative pessimistic assessment of the patient's medical condition has been shown to have the same effect. 200 patients with a random variety of subjective symptoms but no physical evidence of illness were randomly assigned to two consultation groups. At the end of 2 weeks, 64% of patients in the positive consultation group announced they were better or improved as compared to only 46% in the negative consultation grouping.(5)

Talk delivers results. Our mind, it appears, reacts to the information it is fed. Recovery is sprung from the hope belief and expectation that recovery will occur. Results in my Ritual spring I have no doubt from my absolute conviction that my Ritual will keep me well.

A BRIEF INSIGHT IN TO WHAT IS HAPPENING IN THE WORLD OF PLACEBO RESEARCH

In 1998 two psychology researchers at the University of Connecticut, Irving Kirsch and Guy Sapirstein considered the therapeutic benefit to patients of taking, any one of a number, of just over 3000 different types of anti – depressants. Their research established that patients did benefit from taking anti-depressants, in that a sometimes significant improvement in symptoms was observed from a variety of anti – depressants including, SSRI's, tricyclics, and MAO inhibitors, (one of the earliest anti-depressants prescribed from the 1950's onwards.)

The shock the research delivered was that those taking dummy anti-depressant medication obtained 75% of the symptom relief delivered by the genuine anti- depressant although they had only taken an inert substance. Three quarters of the benefit of an anti – depressant was delivered by a sugar pill. (6)

Isn't that amazing? A 75% improvement in symptoms as a result of the trick played upon a patient's mind by a man in a white coat handing over a tablet.

The critical factor at work in the anti – depressant studies, says Irving Kirsch, is belief,

" ....*our beliefs about what is going to happen to us. You don't have to rely upon drugs to see profound transformation".*

Placebo medication has been shown to have effect in relieving the urinary symptoms associated with benign prostatic hyperplasia. (7) Two study groups were created, both containing patients with benign prostatic hyperplasia. One group received an active drug, one group a placebo inert alternative made of starch and cornflour. The group receiving the fake medication not only reported an improvement in urinary function and relief of symptoms, but more mysteriously, they also demonstrated a range of side effects that had been predicted may occur, including impotence, nausea, diarrhoea and constipation. Remember they suffered for no reason, no active substance having been given, to cause those in the trial to suffer in any way.

Continue to be amazed.

If the placebo response does not make you gasp at the yet to be unlocked secrets of the mind and its power to direct self healing, consider, 'nocebo', the negative consequences that can result from giving a patient an entirely fake medication, or subjecting a patient to a fake medical procedure together with a prediction of the likely side effects. Remember, in all the documented experiments, what was happening to a patient was a deceit, an invention of facts, put in to the mind of a patient which the patient believed in. All a fake!

Nothing is really happening to a patient but the disastrously negative impact of the 'nocebo response'. Whether 'nocebo' is demonstrated by a headache, induced by telling a patient a fake electrical current is to be passed through his or her brain, or hair loss resulting from a false declaration that hair loss is likely to occur as a result of swallowing a tablet that is made of sugar but said to be chemotherapy, 'nocebo' consequences are real.

Nocebo is self- directed, self harm, resulting from the direction of our body by our mind. It is not a necessary consequence of a sugar pill or surgery that is make believe. Sugar and theatricals cannot cause harm but our brains can as a result of the information they receive, process and believe in.

Which rather than terrifying is exciting and inspirational news.

If it is little to do with the substance of a procedure or a pill and all to do with our expectation and belief as to what a tablet or procedure can deliver we can invent our own procedures. It is what I have done. I have invented a daily Ritual and brainwashed or conditioned myself in to believing in its therapeutic results, and it has worked.

A friend of mine suggested my Ritual pattern of exercises is indistinguishable from a therapy which involves wearing a purple hat while eating a banana and believing that all ills will be cured. That is, as my friend correctly points out, my Ritual can have no bio-chemical power in itself, there is no reason it has to be in the form it presently is. It could according to my friend be any one of a dozen invented rituals.

I believe she is right, apart from one obvious fact. My Ritual has as much bio chemical power as corn starch! It is a competitor for the placebo pill. It delivers effects whether by wrapping up all aspects of my present boundless energy and perfect health in one placebo effect or by other more significant means.

I have also learned along the way that it is not so much the component parts of my Ritual that are relevant but the manner in which my Ritual is acted out, the platform it has and the elements combined within its performance.

But I digress, let us get back to what is happening in the world of placebo experiment.

Sophisticated scanning techniques now available in modern medicine allow the brain to be observed to establish what is happening when a patient is given a 'dummy' placebo medication or subjected to a 'sham' surgical procedure.

Some of the most exciting research conducted in the field of placebo science has been carried out at the University of Turin by Fabrizio Benedetti and his team. Fabrizio Benedetti has studied the impact of placebo analgesia on the brain and has also conducted work with Parkinson's patients believing, ' the most productive models to understand the neurobiology of the placebo effect are pain and Parkinson's disease.' (8). Benedetti describes the placebo effect as a psychosocial context effect. He suggests the words and rituals of medicine may change the chemistry and circuitry in a patient's brain. The work of Benedetti demonstrates the same biochemical pathways used by opiates such as marijuana and opium are triggered by placebo analgesia, which, Benedetti concludes, suggests there is a cognitive aspect to a drug's success.

Placebo trials carried out with Parkinson's patients show a placebo dopamine tablet, devoid of dopamine, has the power to significantly increase dopamine levels within the brains of Parkinson's sufferers when sufferers believed there was a 75% chance of an active drug being given to them. The expectation, of a 75% chance of receiving an active drug, triggered the patient's reward system, which the scientists conducting the trial felt was essential to triggering a placebo effect. (9)

In 2004 a strong placebo response was demonstrated by a group of patients suffering from Parkinson's disease involved in a double blind trial conducted to establish the success of a sham surgical procedure as compared to a medical transplant of human embryonic dopamine neurons. The trial considered the quality of life of patients in the year after the real and sham transplant procedure. In every case where patients believed they had received a genuine transplant better quality of life scores were recorded even if the patient assessing the quality of his or her life had received nothing. (10)

MAGIC TRICKERY OR DECEIT

Placebo scientists have time and again demonstrated that sham events of surgery can deliver as effective symptom relief as actual surgery involving blood and knives. The ethics of carrying out such fake events of surgery are a matter of philosophical and medical debate but the undoubted information gained about what causes the body to heal is invaluable.

As long ago as 1959 a young surgeon Leonard Cobb made nonsense of an established surgical technique to deal with symptoms of angina in heart patients. (11) The accepted surgical repair technique was to treat angina by effectively knotting and tethering together two arteries. Leonard Cobb doubted the surgical efficacy of the long used technique. He tested the procedure in a series of operations in which he did not knot the arteries. The patient's involved believed they were to receive the standard procedure but Leonard Cobb did not perform the operation, he simply made a series of small incisions in the patient's chest to persuade the patient something had been done.

Despite the artifice 80 % of patients undergoing the 'fake' surgery substantially improved doing as well as those undergoing the full surgical technique.

In 1994 a surgeon named Bruce Moseley conducted a trial using a sham surgical procedure on a group of patients to allow medics to consider the therapeutic benefits to patients of arthroscopy. This is a surgical procedure involving the scraping and rinsing of the knee joint to alleviate symptoms of chronic knee pain. Ten patients were involved in the trial, two underwent full arthroscopy, three had their knee joint rinsed but not scraped and five had nothing at all but a jab in the knee with a scalpel while sedated, to create the effect that surgery had occurred.(12)

Six months after surgery, the ten patients all reported improvement in symptoms of chronic knee pain, with those undergoing the sham procedure reporting an equal improvement in symptoms. No one patient knew if they had received fake surgery or not. The startling fact for the economists in charge of budgets for any national health service is that doing nothing to a patient's knee produced the same level of symptom improvement as an established and supposedly effective surgical procedure.

Real surgical procedures must compete with a trick of surgical repair to allow continual assessment of the merits of any one surgical technique.

The sham surgery trials demonstrate to me a type of 'magic' in the healing potential of the body.

I believe understanding something of the complexity of the placebo response and something of what is happening in the world of placebo research is a means of changing the way we all think about our own health, our body and our mind and more importantly the degree of responsibility we each must accept for the shape we are in, and the quality of life we possess.

Some trial results when I first came across them were so evidently straight from a magician's box of tricks that I almost overlooked the fact that they were evidence of another kind of magic, that is not magic at all but an expression of our innate gift for self repair.

Disappearing warts tested my credibility to the limit.

It was in a trial in 1991 conducted by Jerome Frank at the John Hopkins University in the United States that warts disappeared. (13) Warts suffered by a patient were painted with a brightly coloured dye. Patients within the trial were told the warts would disappear as the dye wore off. The effect of the harmless dye in causing the warts to reduce in size and vanish was as effective as surgical excision of similar warts. It is reported that patients expected their warts to disappear with the fake treatment they were given and they did!

IS IT ALL IN THE MIND?

Asthmatics breathe more effectively after taking a sugar pill. It should be headline news don't you think? But it is more complicated than that, the same asthmatics are also made considerably worse by a device containing nothing but fresh air.

In medical trialling involving asthma patients a placebo medication has been seen to act, both as a bronchodilator, aiding respiration, and a respiratory depressant, inducing a difficulty in breathing; the beneficial or detrimental outcome dependent upon the description given to a patient, by a doctor, of the drug's expected pharmacological effect.

Do you not find that extraordinary?

You may not be asthmatic but in every other respect you are the same as a participant in this placebo trial. You are human with the same structures within your brain and the same structures within your body. You have the same reasoning mind as the asthmatic candidates tricked in to breathing more efficiently. They received nothing at all from the medical men. The reaction within their lungs they created for themselves as a consequence of information received and processed by the brain.

Something happens to evoke a placebo response. Do you see that? Do you see why I believe in the Ritual I perform? Why I obtain the health benefits I obtain?

Or not? Perhaps I just feel in good shape. Perhaps I act as a significantly younger man because I am deceiving myself. So what! Is my response to that. As long as I can power down a wave on my windsurfer, or take my first leap across the sea on my kite surfing board, or make sure I never have to live in a care home or become dependent on any one to toilet me, what does it matter if, ' it is all in my mind ?'

And it could be, a further recent placebo trial, (14) again involving asthmatics shows that even though patients receiving placebo medications believed they had improved, there was no physiological objective evidence to confirm that they had. They felt better; they acted like people who felt better, but they were not clinically improved. The respiration rate of the asthmatic patients when measured still showed the same signs of constriction in their airways as they had demonstrated before they had taken the placebo treatment.

So what!! And I am shouting it now. The important thing is, this group of patients were better in the place it really matters, in their head. Like the child divers on the high cliff ledge, they were defeating the reality their body presented, restricted respiratory function, and disability, because of the belief they held within themselves that they could breathe better.

Child divers dive defeating death and asthmatics breathe more effectively than they have in decades because they believe that they can. Who is the medic to intervene and say they are wrong? Is it the role of the medic to produce charts of the physical forces a spine and neck can withstand and the likely velocity and impact that will result from 100 metre fall, to demonstrate objectively the dive that has just been made should lead to paraplegia or death? Or is it the role of the medic to be amazed, to be humble in the face of what can be achieved, once whatever it is that triggers the placebo effect is unleashed.

The latter I feel should be the approach of the 21st century medic if he or she is to develop a sufficient openness of mind to look beyond the charts of forced expiration volume to the reality that asthmatics breathe as deeply as their belief allows.

IS IT NECESSARY TO DECEIVE TO TRIGGER SELF HEALING?

In a placebo trial many patients do not have the full picture. They know they are in a trial but they do not know if they are to receive an active pharmaceutical. In many trials active as opposed to placebo pills are randomly allocated to patients by computer selection, physicians and patients in the trial not aware when a pill is dispensed, whether a real or dummy pill has been allocated.

With sham surgery the deceit is more overt. A pretence of surgery is constructed in order to make a patient 'believe', that surgery has occurred.

In both cases the brain of the patient is deceived. Expectation results. A patient believes the pill or surgical event is the route to a cure and a placebo response is evoked. The patient feels better, disease is beaten or symptomology improved.

If deceit is essential to triggering our mechanism for self repair how can I deceive myself? My Ritual is delivered through my effort in habitually practising a regime which engages my mind as conductor and orchestrator of my good health rather than as a duped fool.

How can my openly administered Ritual stimulate the necessary bio chemical pathways in my brain to engage and drive self –healing, or regeneration of my being?

I agree it would be impossible to deceive my own brain. I can brainwash myself. I believe there is an aspect of brainwashing that underlies the potency of my Ritual, but something else is necessary, something inexplicable which engages my brain in a particular way to work upon my physical self. This is the elusive part; the elusive response, that is wrapped up in the deception of the credulous patient mind, provoking a biological response which my openness could not lead to.

I would be compelled to seek another explanation for my good luck, my vital life and the optimal health my Ritual delivers, if in 2010 further placebo research conducted by Ted Kaptchuk and his team at Harvard, had not turned over another piece, in the placebo jigsaw, which had marked upon it, the words, 'DECEIT NOT REQUIRED'.

This 2010 trial used a cohort of patients troubled by symptoms of irritable bowel syndrome. The trials were unique in that patients were not deceived when given a placebo pill but told in straightforward terms that the group of patients they had been assigned to were to receive placebo pills.

Whatever the nature of the bio-chemical mechanisms that allow the mind to direct the body to heal itself ; it is now demonstrated such mechanisms can still be accessed, even when patients are told the ritual of prescribing they are involved in, is simply role play and not a ritual of prescribing at all. Placebo responses can occur without deception.

In the 2010 trial, one group of patients received no treatment at all, while those in Group 2 were told they would be taking fake inert drugs. The pills were delivered to patients in bottles marked 'placebo pills'.

The patients were told placebos often deliver clinical results and have a healing effect. The patients in Group 2 who accepted the bottle of placebo pills and took the pills knowing they were a fake treatment described a real improvement in their symptoms. The patients in Group 2 obtained twice as much symptom relief as those in the no treatment group. The most remarkable fact was that the level of symptom improvement among IBS sufferers taking a placebo, knowing what they placed in to their mouth was a fake drug, was at the same level as that seen in patients taking the best performing active IBS drugs.

The patients had been told that the tablets were placebos and that placebos could bring symptom relief.

I tell myself every day, my Ritual is working as placebos do, and placebos deliver results because they activate the body to self-heal. Ted Kaptchuk's 2010 trial establishes for me, that the amazing bio-mechanical mechanism within us all that can deliver self healing, can still operate even if my brain is not deceived but aware that I expect to get well, to live longer, to enjoy better health as a result of a Ritual I have invented.

It is important, that anyone reading this book, who decides to give my Ritual a go, appreciates one very important point.

When the Ritual is begun there need not be complete conviction or belief that the Ritual will work, but there must be some sense from the first session onwards that some benefit will be gained from the practice. Even a minimal shift in perspective from outright cynicism to an acceptance of the remote likelihood of results will suffice, because the Ritual will produce its own beneficial results and be in a sense, self serving.

As the results of the Ritual are delivered and witnessed through improving health, changed outlook, lessening lethargy, or symptom reduction in any ill the body has, the mind will be persuaded that the Ritual delivers results. Self-healing, self maintenance, self rejuvenation will become the expected outcome of every Ritual session, and through belief in outcome, do not ask me why, outcome will be realised.

IS MY RITUAL AHEAD OF ITS TIME?

I am aware that many of the trial results I have set down were obtained many years ago. I have run through the results I found most astounding the first time I came across them but I do not want anyone to think research effort into decoding placebo is not ongoing, or not daily producing new information to take us onwards, towards an understanding of the healing power we all possess.

I am outside the world of placebo science. I like to read the conclusion of trials and tests involving placebos. I get lost in the minutiae of the science but my mind leaps on facts that demonstrate the magical ability we all have within us to defy conventional expectation of our potential. Cyclists told they had been given a powerful caffeine laced tablet, cycle faster, and out do their, 'personal best' timings, when they have been given nothing at all. New York commuters segregated in to three groups and given, painkiller, versus placebo, versus nothing, to deal with an early morning headache surprise everyone by curing head pain with a tablet as chemically effective as fresh air.

I love to hear that. I am an optimist. I am optimistic about the potential we all have to self-maintain and self-repair without the crushing weight of the drug industry bearing down upon us with yet another shovel load of the latest bio-chemicals.

I want Ted Kaptchuk, and Irving Kirsch, and Fabrizio Benedetti to complete their life's work now. I want it to be explained in textbooks made available to every medical student how our mechanism to engage with illness, to recalibrate our organism towards health, can be engaged.

I am sure mankind will get there but I don't have the patience to wait until those who merit them receive the necessary research grants and peer support to do their work.

I am seventy years old with a life to lead and I want to live it well.

If I had the guide book, that I know will be written, to explain why fake medicines and procedures heal, and a second volume telling me how I could apply what placebo science reveals about self healing to my own life I would buy both books and use them.

I would have no need to write this book to explain how, inspired by the world of placebo science and the potential for self-healing placebos reveal, I created a Ritual that has effectively changed every aspect of my life, and in its working, has kept me well, and dramatically slowed the rate at which I am appearing to age.

CHAPTER THREE

TRIGGERS

What triggers self -healing and the placebo response?

That is a really big question. Knowing the answer to this question is akin to handing to every being on this earth the gift of eternal life.

So who knows?

No one!!!

It is important to remember that, because it is the truth, as it stands today, on this Wednesday, in this month, at this point, in the history of mankind, not one scientist has perfectly worked out what it is that triggers the placebo response, or what I prefer to term, our ability to self-heal.

There is, in the medical and scientific literature, much debate, but no definitive position. There is speculation upon the brain's engagement with hope, expectation and reward. There is talk of conditioning; discussion upon the theatricals of medicine, and the power of white coats and stethoscopes. There is inter-discipliniary effort made to engage. Philosophers meeting with biologists, physicists crossing the divide to confront the power in 'energy' therapies. There is, in modern science, an ongoing quest to understand what in the psychology, or physiology of a human can possibly explain the potential of our body to self-repair.

The science of placebo is still emerging, and I am still learning. Let us take a look at the debate. Let's see what the greatest in the field of placebo science think the trigger of the placebo response could be. This trigger once identified is, I believe, the trigger to self –healing. It is the secret revealed that explains why physiological, bio- chemical change occurs within the body when nothing is swallowed but a sugar pill and nothing is performed but a Ritual invented by an average man in search of a longer, healthier life.

THEORY NO 1:

A CONDITIONED RESPONSE

When you walk in to a doctor's waiting room you begin to feel better. Have you noticed that? Have you noticed how, perhaps for the first time in days, the symptoms you are experiencing do not seem as acute?

It is said we react not only to medicine but to the environment of medicine. We are conditioned, by previous outcomes delivered by a doctor's intervention, to associate visiting a doctor with recovery and so we feel better.

Stethoscopes, anatomy charts, the smell of antiseptic, can, it is said, by those promoting classical conditioning theory, to explain the triggering of a placebo response, prompt symptom improvement or healing.

Healing for the classical conditioning theorists is bound up with a learned association in the mind of the patient between what should be the neutral stimulus of a doctor's consulting room, which can of itself deliver nothing to the patient, and a physiological result. The patient self heals or symptoms improve because, it is said, the patient associates the symbols of healing with healing itself. Past association made between the healing symbols, sounds and smells, within a doctor's consultation room and recovery are enough to elicit a response in the body as a result of the cognitive processes of association and learning.

Classical conditioning theory is known to many of us as a result of the work of Russian scientist Ivan Pavlov. The expression 'Pavlov's Dog', has become the term most frequently used to describe a learned response. It comes from an experiment conducted by Ivan Pavlov in 1927 to study a learned response in a dog to what otherwise should have been a neutral event.

Ivan Pavlov demonstrated that dogs could be made to salivate at the ringing of a bell, in the same way they did at feeding time, even though no actual food was produced or seen. Pavlov rang a bell every time the dogs were fed. Eventually through learning and association the dogs salivated simply at the ringing of the bell without any food being seen or given to them. Pavlov concluded that the brain of the dog responded in a learned rather than intuitive way, delivering a physiological response to a stimulus that should not of itself have been capable of producing a response.

The brain of the dog ultimately responded to a bell in the same way it had originally responded to food. The analogy being that if an association is made between the environment of medicine and healing, a patient can ultimately trigger healing in the body simply by being exposed to the environment of medicine alone.

What do you think about that?

You sit with a doctor ; he gives you a pill. Presumably a real pill with real pharmacological potential and you heal? What did it? - the pill; or your past association with the process of medicine?

Hard to know many doctors would concede. Doctors have even admitted to prescribing 'placebo' drugs in circumstances where they knew the drug given was likely to have little clinical benefit simply to satisfy the demand a patient makes, for a medicine, for something to carry away, to allow the process of recovery to begin.

I applied the tenets of classical conditioning to my Ritual. Was I conditioning myself to respond to a Ritual, by reinforcing in my brain the certain fact that the procedure I followed every morning was health inducing? Can we condition, or effectively 'brainwash' ourselves in the absence of third party participation? Can the brain be 'fooled' in the same way by auto- conditioning to trigger the body's indisputable ability to self -heal.

In my case what is making me feel as good as I do? My active engagement with my Ritual or an alternative process of the brain analogous to that fired when a placebo drug is given which prompts the mechanism of self –healing?

Is my programme, my act of performance of my Ritual every morning, allocating time, using a dedicated 'therapy' space created within my home, creation of a meditative state of mind, repetition of the same pattern of touch and movement, sufficient in itself to convert what should be a neutral event, something many say is without therapeutic value, in to a healing mechanism?

If the effectiveness of my Ritual in delivering consequences for my health and wellbeing is a result of some type of auto conditioning at what point did I become conditioned and so associate my Ritual with health? I asked myself that and the obvious answer came to me.

From the outset of performance I believed in the efficacy of my Ritual. From the day it was first constructed I believed by dedicating myself to the pattern of actions my Ritual demanded I would improve my health. I knew there was enough therapeutic potential in the Ritual I had invented for results to be delivered. I could not say, of what type, whether gain would be physiological or psychological but I did believe results of some sort, change of some sort would be the consequence of incorporating the therapeutic Ritual I had constructed in to my life. I knew at an instinctive level results would come. I 'knew', because I believed I had created my own placebo and that my Ritual would work as effectively as a sugar pill. My reasoning was no more complicated than that. My belief in my early Ritual may seem risible, but there it is, inspired by what was happening in placebo science, I believed.

Within weeks I felt differently. If asked to explain how I felt, I would say, 'better than I had', 'the same but more alive'.

Was that the point at which I had become conditioned? The point at which the moment I lay down in my dedicated performance space the therapeutic benefits of my Ritual began to be felt? I undoubtedly associated my good health with performance of my set of ritualistic actions. To feel good I needed only to make time, create space, position myself for my Ritual to begin and a host of positive emotions flooded in to me. Calmness, optimism, expectancy; settling myself for my Ritual to begin meant whatever was troubling me, whatever negative emotion I was carrying, dissipated.

Just like sitting down in a chair in the Doctor's waiting room induces calm in many a mind, my Ritual induces calm and a sense of wellbeing in me. Whatever state I am in I feel better when my Ritual begins. Health, wellbeing, and the performance of my Ritual are now inextricably linked in my mind.

If I am conditioned I am conditioned, call it what you will. But auto-conditioning cannot be the whole answer to the success my Ritual has had. There was inevitably a point before habitual performance induced in me certain expectations of therapeutic benefit. The first time I began my Ritual I could not be conditioned to expect results, as my Ritual had not shown what it could do.

The early results, the first changes came in any event. Before they were demonstrable there was a space of days or weeks when something else was going on. Something other than conditioning caused the first improvements in my health to occur something which conditioning now probably overlays.

What classical conditioning theory does demonstrate to me is the importance of context and the association the brain makes between environment and outcome. Setting has an emotional aspect to it and emotions affect the activity of the mind. The setting in which a therapy is delivered matters. The ritual of performance matters, both are effective at conditioning the mind to perceive a certain result will occur.

THEORY NO 2:

EXPECTATION:

Expecting a particular result causes the brain to fire in a particular way to deliver the result expected.

I will go with that.

I am entirely committed to my Ritual. I expect my daily performance to deliver results. I constructed it in a way I considered would inevitably do me good and even in the first weeks of performing it I expected it to have an effect upon me which over time would be beneficial. I did not feel any different in the first days of working with my Ritual. I did not look in the mirror and see any tangible difference in my appearance. My Ritual was a good thing to do. I felt that. When I had finished even the first performance of my Ritual I felt calm and relaxed. I felt instinctively that the very act of achieving a relaxed state of mind, stepping out of my usual pattern of thought had been good for me and I wanted to renew the experience to incorporate the Ritual in to my day- to- day life.

Even from initial performance something had been triggered within my brain. I cannot know or scientifically assess if it was a self- healing response but as I reflect on what scientists have demonstrated about the tangible physiological consequences of expectation I marvel at what my Ritual may be able to achieve.

When we expect something good to happen our brains produce dopamine. This has been demonstrated by the experiment involving patients suffering from Parkinson's disease conducted by Jon Stoessl of the University of British Columbia.(1)

Patients suffering symptoms of the disease were injected with a saline solution and were told it was an active medication intended to alleviate symptoms and improve motor control. The patients experienced an improvement in symptoms of tremor and increased motor control and an increase in the level of dopamine in the brain of each patient was documented. This really happened. Intransigent neurological disease was fooled by expectation and defeated. Nothing but a salt solution was given to the ill patients, but they did not know that. They believed they had been given a powerful pharmaceutical able to impact on their brain and the processes within it to increase production of dopamine. They believed relief would come and it did, their dopamine levels increased and they felt better. Salt did it, but not salt alone. Salt and expectation.

My emotional state when I commence my Ritual is one of expectation.

I expected the act of dedicating myself to my Ritual to impact upon my body in a beneficial way.

Is this mind state alone causing me to feel better, my health to improve, my body to rejuvenate?

I have no doubt expectation is powerful. I find it easy to accept that a patient who expects to become well has a more significant chance of achieving wellness than a patient who doubts a cure can be delivered.

But is this why sugar pills, corn- starch and sham surgery all have the power to heal?

Those who present patient expectation as the essential trigger of the placebo response would certainly have us believe so.

Consider this!

It has been demonstrated a group of people given a drink they are told contains strong alcohol are likely to exhibit all the signs of intoxication after drinking only one or two glasses even though the drink in their hand has nothing in it but flavoured water. A group given decaffeinated coffee to drink and told it is an ordinary caffeinated brew will demonstrate every physiological consequence of drinking strong caffeinated coffee. Chemotherapy patients after only two chemotherapy sessions with a drug that induces nausea are nauseous simply entering the unit in which they are being treated with out any drug being given to them.

Expectation, is the agent, the stimulant that is processed by the brain prior to the expected result being delivered.

Not surprisingly with such considered potency expectation has been the subject of extensive scientific experiment and study. The many experiments conducted demonstrate the fundamental role patient expectation plays in delivery of a beneficial or indeed destructive outcome.

Chemotherapy patients told their hair may fall out have been shown to suffer hair loss even when the tablets given to them are inert capsules containing nothing that could cause hair loss to occur.

So what is within this emotional state of expectation? What does expectation change? What impact does it have upon the brain to so dramatically affect the outcome of medical treatment?

Well it does something: that has been proven. Walter Brown M.D writing for the Psychiatric Times in 2006 confirmed:

'The results of several brain imaging studies suggest that expectation has a neuroanatomic and neurophysiologic basis'.

Walter Brown goes on to cite the outcome of an experiment involving Parkinson's patients the brains of whom had been implanted with stimulating electrodes. If the electrodes were turned off motor performance diminished and conversely if the electrodes were turned on motor performance improved. Trials demonstrated that a sham turning off procedure when the electrodes remained on resulted in reduced motor performance in any event, if the patient's believed the electrodes had been turned off. Conversely when patients were told electrodes would be turned back on motor performance improved even though the electrodes remained off.

In 1988 Kirsch and Weixel (2) carried out the experiment involving the coffee drinkers. Trial participants were divided in to two groups. One group involved a double blind study of experimenters and trial participants. In this group participants knew they would either receive caffeinated coffee or a decaffeinated substitute but they did not know which. A second group of participants were told they would be served an ordinary caffeinated coffee when in fact decaffeinated coffee was given.

Participants in this second group who anticipated and expected a response from their decaffeinated coffee - that a real coffee would produce- had higher pulse rates, different levels of tension, alertness and systolic blood pressure, than participants in the 'double blind' grouping. It was determined that the higher pulse rates etc. correlated with the higher level of expectation of effects from the coffee within the second grouping, as opposed to the more equivocal expectation of those in the first group, not fully knowing if decaffeinated or caffeinated coffee had been given.

I emphasise those in Group 2 demonstrated, clear, objectively assessable, signs of drinking strong coffee, which resulted from nothing more than their expectation of those effects. Those in Group 1 did not know what to expect. They did not know what they were to receive and so expectation could not play a certain role in their responses; hence argue the placebo scientists, the potential for a demonstrable placebo response was less.

I have already discussed the meta analysis of anti-depressant medication carried out by Irving Kirsch et al in 2008. The difference in effect of placebo anti-depressants compared to active drug anti-depressants was found to be small even in some cases where patients were severely depressed. Moreover the only difference in effectiveness between a drug and a placebo was due to the efficacy of a placebo diminishing with repeated administration rather than the efficacy of the anti-depressant increasing.

Irving Kirsch discussed his work on anti-depressants and his findings about their clinical effectiveness at an *International Research Conference on Integrative Medicine and Health* in Portland Oregon in 2012. He presented conference delegates with the results of his work that demonstrated that anti-depressants when used in cases of mild to moderate depression, have no statistically measurable effect. Subsequently interviewed about this conclusion he stated.

'*Emotions, expectancies, and behavioural conditioning like that of Pavlov's dog have long been known to affect the body. This is the basis of the placebo effect. Timothy Walsh has done a meta-analysis on the effects of placebo and drugs over time. He showed that as public awareness of anti-depressants increased the response to drugs and placebos for depression also increased.*'

When interviewed by CBS news about the same body of work, Kirsch was even clearer. When asked if sugar pills create the same effects as anti-depressants, Kirsch replied;

"They'd have almost as large an affect, and whatever difference it would be, would be clinically insignificant.... people get better when they take the drug, but it's not the chemical ingredients of the drugs that are making them better, it's largely the placebo effect"

In *The Science of the Placebo: Toward an Interdisciplinary Research Agenda (3);* the following comment is made about the trials conducted by Kirsch & Saperstein :

'Results of placebo controlled clinical trials of antidepressants generally show small or no differences between active drug and placebo. As a result of a meta-analysis of studies of antidepressant medications, these investigators suggest that antidepressant drugs may be little more than active placebos that reinforce patients' response expectancies in so far as they produce side effects'.

Which if you think about it, is incredible. The drug companies are making literally millions of dollars from the sale of antidepressants and yet the pills they sell need not make a patient well to make a patient well. Instead a medicine need only create an impact within the body, that is a side effect of itself, for the patient to believe something is happening and so expect and believe in a cure; which as a result of triggering something, still elusive within us, results in the cure expected.

So is expectation the answer?

Is my expectation that my Ritual will deliver results enough to manifest the results I am witnessing?

Is expectation the true trigger of self- healing within us?

What then of conditioning? Is it a separate trigger or part and parcel of expectation?

Complicated isn't it? Well this is a massive area of science. The facts are still emerging and the stakes are high. If science solves the mystery of what the trigger is that flicks the switch inside us that allows self healing to begin, why would we ever be ill, and more outrageous than even that startling proposition, why would we ever die, if the alternative was continual repair?

So yes it is complicated, but perhaps in accepting the hidden trigger is not one single mechanism but a complex device with many levers within it we move one step closer to identifying what really is the key to our perpetual wellness.

THEORY 3

IT'S COMPLICATED

Richard Bootzin a psychologist from the University of Arizona accepts that. Richard Bootzin contributed to the conference held in 2000 to decode placebo and in the BMJ publication resulting from the conference papers Richard Bootzin offers the opinion that we cannot seek to isolate any one trigger of self healing within us if we are to get any closer to solving the placebo puzzle.

His view is reported as follows;

'the placebo effect is not static, but a dynamic, constantly changing variable, co- varying with other variables, both psychological and physiological, that operate within the therapeutic process. The interactions are not predictable but operate synergistically with the active treatment (rather than simply adding to active treatment effects). He emphasizes that the meaning ascribed by the patient to the health problem and the treatment proposed provides a context in which a number of mechanisms may operate- conditioning, expectancies, information from the clinician, internal feedback- with reciprocal and recursive interactions' (4)

That's a long way of saying, IT'S COMPLICATED.

Bootzin tells me the 'meaning' I ascribe to my Ritual performance is important in creating an appropriate context in which self- healing may occur. I do imbue my Ritual with huge significance. To me the daily practice of my Ritual has become synonymous with lasting health. To me my daily performance means I will stay well, live longer, look better and live a better life. I could not, if I tried, imbue my Ritual with any greater meaning for my life and so I wanted to look a little further at what the impact of giving meaning to a process achieves. Could meaning in itself be the trigger?

THEORY 4.

PLACEBO RESPONSE OR MEANING RESPONSE.

It should not even be called the placebo response. The results obtained from sugar pills should be seen as a response to the meaning the pill has for the patient in the trial. This conclusion comes from the work of Daniel E. Moerman, Phd, and Wayne B. Jonas MD who believe we should look at the placebo response in a different way to that in which it has been considered over many years.

Daniel Moerman and Wayne Jonas in their paper I have already referred to entitled; *Deconstructing the Placebo Effect and Finding the Meaning Response,(5)* remind us that placebos can- not cause the placebo effect, they cannot cause any thing, they are inert pills. It is said we should consider things differently and look at the placebo response in terms of patients responding to the meaning and significance they find in any particular therapy.

Two experiments are discussed, the first involving medical students asked to participate in a study of two drugs, one a stimulant, one a tranquilizer. Each student was given a packet containing one or two blue or red tablets. Following tablet use the students were asked to complete questionnaires to describe the effect of the pills taken. The questionnaires gave the common opinion of the students that the blue tablets acted as depressants while the red tablets acted as stimulants and in all cases taking two tablets produced a greater effect than taking one tablet.

A second study involved 835 British women who regularly suffered from headaches. The women were randomly assigned to one of four groups. One group received aspirin labelled with a widely advertised brand name, a brand that had been popular and widely used in the UK for many years. A second group received the same tablet in a plain box. The third group received a placebo tablet in a plain packet and the fourth group received a placebo tablet marked with the same widely advertised brand name. Results obtained demonstrated, branded aspirin worked better than unbranded, which worked better than branded placebo, which worked better than unbranded placebo.

The branded placebo relieved a headache and branded painkillers worked best of all, hence the plea of those going to the GP to give them the medicine they usually get, not one of those, 'generic substitutes'.

The inevitable conclusion; people respond not to a particular medicine but to the meaning they give to a medicine. Moerman and Jonas define this meaning response as:

'the physiologic or psychological effects of meaning in the origins or treatment of illness; meaning responses elicited after the use of inert or sham treatment can be called the 'placebo effect' when they are desireable and the 'nocebo effect' when they are undesireable'.

For Moerman and Jonas medicine is permeated with meaning. They cite the physician's white coat, the stethoscope, the presentment of a diagnosis, the manner of announcement of a prognosis.

The meaning a patient gives to a sugar pill taken can have substantial physiological consequences. Moerman provides us with the example of placebo analgesia. Scientific experiment has demonstrated a sugar pill given as a pain -killer causes the body to produce and release endorphins, the body's natural pain relieving bio chemicals.

Moerman concludes his paper with the following enquiry.

'......, a huge puzzle remains: Obviously the meaning response is of great value to the sick and the lame. For example, eliciting the meaning response requires remarkably little effort ("You will be fine, Mr Smith"). So why does this not happen all the time? And why can't you do it for yourself?'

I hold my breath, and await science answering the question, because I am doing just that. I am eliciting in my body a response to the Ritual I have created, in part, I am certain, because of the meaning I have imbued my Ritual with.

I can therefore, 'do it for myself ', is the answer I would give.

In their paper, and I do not know if their views have changed, Daniel Moerman and Wayne Jonas respond in a different way:

'Perhaps only when a friend, relative, or healer indicates some level of social support, (for example, by performing a ritual) is the individual's internal economy able to act'.

Who is right? Must I get somebody in to perform a ritual if I want my body to heal itself, or has my body got it right in getting on with the job for itself?

THEORY 5

THE RITUAL OF MEDICINE

The Navajo certainly get somebody in. In fact they get in a whole cast of characters and props and scenery to create a ritual for healing a member of their tribe that has been described by Ted Kaptchuk as, 'the equivalent of a Wagnerian Opera'.

In his paper entitled : *Placebo Studies and Ritual Theory: a comparative analysis of Navajo, acupuncture and biomedical healing.* (6) Ted Kaptchuk looks at the rituals involved in healing and what they tell us about the placebo response.

Ted Kaptchuk considers ritual healing has an impact on the symptoms of an illness, not simply by altering the manner in which symptoms are considered by the patient but by altering neurobiological mechanisms within the patient who is ill. He concludes, *'placebo effects are the 'specific' effects of healing rituals.'*

Ted Kaptchuk compares Navajo Indian healing ceremonies involving chant pathways, to Chinese acupuncture and to every day bio- medical medicine, offered when we visit a GP.

The rituals although from entirely different cultures and acted out in entirely different ways have much in common in that they provide a context in which healing can occur.

There is a type of theatre in each of the rituals considered. The Navajo ceremonies are the most elaborate. Tribal stories of wrong- doing and redemption are acted out and performed by a cast of many chanting costumed characters. The stories of healing and redemption from antiquity are made relevant to the subject who is ill. The ceremony is supervised by the healer or medicine man who directs the process of the healing.

The theatre of acupuncture is a room filled with, *'acupuncture charts and manikins, Asian art -work and Chinese herbs'*. The ritual is of the insertion of needles in accordance with energy meridians charted over thousands of years.

Ted Kaptchuk makes the point that just as the Navajo healing ceremony connects the small and insignificant person who is to be healed with a greater world of ancient truths so the actions of the acupuncturist, links, as Kaptchuk says, *' the patient's condition to meteorological and macrocosm forces and connects the patient to a wider world of coherent and intentional forces.'*

Mainstream medicine as we have seen is full of ritual.

I would recommend to everyone who has bought this book that they read the entire paper Kaptchuk has produced, not only for the elegance of the way in which Kaptchuk describes the rituals and processes involved in bio-medical healing, which should become a classic description in itself and an aide to remembering what we subject ourselves to when we make that first GP appointment, but also for the conclusion Kaptchuk draws about the impact of the ritual of modern medicine in the process of healing. He writes,

'like the Navajo and acupuncture healing, the biomedical treatment fuses universal forces (which are described in scientific terms) onto a single person's unique suffering.'

I describe in Chapter 5 the process of my Ritual. Rituals, in my opinion, are essential to triggering bodily and mental repair. The very act of participating in a Ritual changes, I believe, the manner in which we consider the being that we are, the state we are in, the perception we have of the body we inhabit, the manner in which we, without an intervening medic, are able to connect to forces within and beyond ourself.

Kaptcuk believes the nearest modern medicine comes to studying the impact of rituals is in the scientific experiments carried out to study the power of placebos. Kaptchuk quotes a medical study in which diazepam, (valium), was given to a patient without the patient knowing. The drug was given, with out the patient being aware. It was in the patient's system, but it had no effect on the patient's post-operative anxiety level until it was given overtly, accompanied by the ritual of a medical professional handing the tablet over in a medical setting. This suggests Kaptchuk demonstrates that ritual is an, *'active component of biomedical treatment'*.

Fabrizio Benedetti, is reported to have written that rituals and drugs use the very same bio-chemical pathways to influence a patient's brain.

The following is said to have been included within an email sent by Benedetti:

'What we 'placebo neuroscientists'...have learned [is] that therapeutic rituals move a lot of molecules in the patients' brain, and these molecules are the very same, as those activated by the drugs we give in routine clinical practice. In other words, rituals and drugs use the very same biochemical pathways to influence the patient's brain' (7)

I knew about shamanic healing when I invented my own Ritual but it never crossed my mind at that time that modern medicine is full of its own rituals and that my own Ritual has echoes within it of a healing ceremony I subject my body to on a daily basis.

I could not now perform my Ritual in any other way than that I describe and set out in great detail in Chapter 5. The manner in which I move my hands and apply pressure to my body, the sequence of actions I carry out, the accompanying visualisation, statement and affirmation is what works. I cannot alter one aspect, as if to alter anything would presage some crippling tattoo or break the enchantment of my created spell.

I am stuck with my Ritual as it is. The Ritual I have invented from nothing has now invested itself with power. Or I believe that it has, which is where we came in, and from where we will head out. The final theory that has been presented to me to explain what triggers the power of placebo is that placebo healing is triggered by a patient's belief. Belief is the most powerful agent of all, it can stand alone or it can raise up and carry upon its back every other theory and explanation given to explain the body's ability to heal itself, for without this one mental state, my Ritual and sugar pills would have no ability to trigger any therapeutic consequence. I believe that.

THEORY 6

THE POWER OF BELIEF:

Belief heals. Any good catholic will tell you that. Catholics know the strongest form of belief any human being can have, blind faith, in a desired outcome, can provide a cure. Catholics believe in miracles and why wouldn't they? Cures that are medically inexplicable in terms of medical treatments and techniques available at the time the cure was delivered have been witnessed 69 times between 1858 and 2013 at the shrine of Our Lady of Lourdes. 69 people with crippling disabilities have been cured instantaneously and permanently, of significantly disabling symptoms, including blindness, after bathing in or drinking the waters of the shrine at Lourdes, or by simply lying down on the ground in the vicinity of the sacred place.

The cures have been verified as cures inexplicable in terms of what was current in medical science at the time the cure was delivered by the *International Medical Committee of Lourdes* after consideration of all patient medical records, (available from patient files held in hospitals and medical centres) which document the original diagnosis of the condition to be 'cured' and the treatment offered by mainstream medicine. The afflictions cured are many and diverse and include the most serious of medical conditions including paralysis and tumours.

Would these 'cures' have been possible without unshakeable faith in the beneficence of an unseen deity? Is faith the most extreme form of belief that can be demonstrated?

Even avoiding an ascent to the centre of the spiritual or a consideration of the power of the worshipped unseen Virgin as opposed to the power of an individual's mind, the answer is probably 'no'. The one component all 'cures' listed in the register of the Medical Bureau of Lourdes have in common is the geography of the shrine. For every recipient of a miracle, the act of positioning the ill person, beside or close to, the shrine, was a pre-requisite of a cure being delivered. Whatever else those cured believed in, each one, prior to receiving deliverance from their disability, firmly believed by visiting Lourdes, healing would occur, or *sine qua non* their individual journeys, often made in arduous circumstances and with all the disadvantages of extreme disability would not have been made.

In the brain of the 69 pilgrims cured I suggest a very definite association between the deliverance of health and the silent pleas that could only be made at the shrine at Lourdes. There was no half –heartedness on the part of the pilgrims. No remaining at home, cosy in bed, with a prayer book in their hand.

All cured were afflicted by massive disability. The long journey they each made was a demonstration of belief. For each of these 69 very ill beings their belief would certainly have been reinforced by their ritual of travelling to the shrine. Inevitably their hope of a cure would have grown stronger as the physical geography of the shrine, (the cave in which, at Lourdes in 1858, the Virgin Mary had appeared to a 14 year old girl), grew near. The presence of other pilgrims, the stories of miracles already delivered must inevitably have strengthened the belief each carried in their mind that their cure would be delivered.

I would suggest at the moment their individual prayers were answered a neurologist able to study what was happening in the brain of each pilgrim would have been able to identify patterns of activity startlingly identical and would, if he or she had been carrying a hand-held scanner, have viewed 69 perfect images of what unshakeable belief looks like when it is formed in the brain.

The firing of neurons in a certain sequence and the massive consequences for the 69 bodies healed cannot be considered, in my opinion, something, only the religious or the devout should be interested in. The blind do see as a result of visiting Lourdes, it is documented. The crippled do walk and throw away their wheelchairs. It is not Galilee at the time of Christ, it is rural France and the last verified healing considered to be inexplicable in terms of current medical science was verified on the 20th June 2013.

Why would the entire world not be interested in that?

Ted Kaptchuk go now, Irving put down your notebooks, Fabrizio Benedetti, you are closer in Turin than either of the other two, I urge you all to go now, immediately, to Lourdes and consider there at the waters near to the shrine, what is the trigger of the placebo effect?

What role does belief play when the task is to heal ourselves?

If there is any one location at which the role of belief in the healing process may be revealed to science it is surely by observation at the shrine.

Is belief in outcome the one essential trigger that makes healing occur?

Can we harness and apply to our life the benefits of belief?

Catholics, and I mean no offence, genuinely believe the sacred Virgin Mary intervenes to eradicate illness and restore health. I believe my Ritual delivers longevity and promotes enduring health. Would my brain, if scanned as my Ritual commences, demonstrate the same patterns of light and dark, of electricity and neural activity, that would be shown on the scans of pilgrims? Is belief alone enough to trigger the neurological consequence of wellness?

If in the years to come it is established as a fact that belief is enough to trigger self-healing I will be satisfied for I have literally brainwashed myself to believe in the benefits of my Ritual. My results may be less dramatic than the cures achieved at Lourdes, but they are tangible, and with great humility I propose, in the most dilute of forms, there is a correlation between my homespun act and the purported intervention of the divine. The modest correlation, being the ability of my mind, to form and hold an unshakeable belief in the outcome of my action, just as a pilgrim does.

I turn now from the mystical to the tragic. The case I report is cited in many commentaries and text- books that deal with mind -body healing. This case demonstrates to me the darker side of belief.

Belief raises us up and carries us and makes manifest what we believe in. Take away a person's belief and watch decimation occur, a spirit collapse, a life spiral inwards to a place that is our destination when hope is lost. I can only imagine the poignancy of the very different electrical activity that would be witnessed on our held scanner of the brain when belief is taken or extinguished by facts revealed.

What is it that happens to the mind when we believe we are to die, that can take our will to live away, causing us to die, when we may not even be ill?

The case of Mr Wright and the trialled cancer drug *Krebiozen* does not fully answer the question but it illustrates both the potency of belief and the consequent devastation likely to occur when belief is removed.

The *Krebiozen* case was used in a paper presented at a conference in 1957 by the US Psychiatrist Bruno Klopfer. Researchers in Bruno Klopfer's clinic were trialling a new cancer drug *Krebiozen*. Mr Wright wanted to try it; when he requested the drug he presented with the advanced stages of lymphosarcoma. At the point he was allowed to commence *Krebiozen* Mr Wright's cancer had demonstrated it was resistant to all other available treatments. Mr Wright was enthusiastic about the prospects of being included within the Krebiozen trial and the drug was given to him although he was not expected to respond to it. At the point it was given he had already developed significant tumour masses in his neck, groin, chest and abdomen. The tumours were considered too advanced to be affected in any way by *Krebiozen.*

The medical team were wrong. After one injection of the drug the witnessed tumours began to shrink and within ten days of treatment commencing Mr Wright was in full remission and had returned to his hobby of flying.

Reports of the efficacy of the drug started circulating and all reports indicated the drug did not work. This news had a severe effect on Mr Wright, his cancer reappeared and his health deteriorated. Aware of what was happening Bruno Klopfer MD tried to intervene, he told his patient a further new strain of *Krebiozen* was now available with much greater potency than the first and he persuaded Mr Wright to take it. Not only was no new drug available but Bruno Klopfer on this second occasion injected Mr Wright with only water. It is documented that Mr Wright's, *'recovery from his second near terminal state was even more dramatic than his first'*. Mr Wright remained symptom free for two months until over whelming negative publicity in the press about *Krebiozen* persuaded him the drug was useless. Within a few days of the press reports rubbishing the drug Mr Wright was readmitted to hospital and within two days he died.

The medical state Mr Wright was in correlated with the state of belief he held about the likely outcome of his treatment. His life or death depended ultimately not upon drugs but upon the nature of his belief. Other examples exist in medical journals of patients offered a diagnosis of cancer said to be terminal only to find at post mortem examination, following inevitably accelerated death, that no malignant mass existed within the patient's tissues sufficient to have caused death to occur. Death, in such cases, results from diagnosis, rather than from disease, or in a nutshell, from belief.

And belief can be based upon the most incredible of facts and still be therapeutic. The Navajo healing ceremonies mentioned previously are in many senses ridiculous. They involve the wild chanting and dancing of costumed performers shaking sticks and enacting rage and redemption as the story of the ill patient is aligned with acts of adultery and revenge taken from stories handed down through Navajo history. Star gazing is a principal means of diagnosis in Navajo traditional medicine. How can such a regime make anyone well? But it does and has done for hundreds of years. A substantial percentage of the Navajo still consult traditional medicine men even though living in the crucible of emerging conventional medical practice, the United States of America. What is healing the Navajo today, their dances, chants and myths, or their belief?

How powerful is belief?

Is it the case that we must be careful what we believe in for it may manifest itself. Is belief equally potent when positive as opposed to negative. If we believe in the health prescription we invent for ourselves can it deliver, whatever its nature, ritual, herbal, or pharmaceutical?

On the 24ᵗʰ October 2013 the following report from journalist Malcolm Moore appeared in the Daily Telegraph. *Cockroach fried twice: China's new 'miracle' drug.* In China in 2013 cockroach farming was on the 'up'. Cockroaches had become popular in China not for their taste but for their medicinal properties. Professor Liu Yusheng at the Shandong agricultural university has announced them to be a 'miracle drug' that really can cure, 'a number of ailments', and 'work much faster than other medicine'. A cream made from powdered cockroaches is used in Chinese hospitals to treat burns while a cockroach syrup invented by a pharmaceutical company in Szechuan promises to cure gastroenteritis, duodenal ulcers and pulmonary tuberculosis.

I think that is enough evidence to persuade us, that just about anything can work if those taking it believe in it.

Undoubtedly something of benefit will be added to the rituals we incorporate in to our daily lives, whether it is swallowing our vitamin pills, bending ourselves in to the most advanced of yoga positions or setting time aside to communicate with our bodies in the way my Ritual demands, if we genuinely believe, a positive therapeutic result will be the outcome.

CHAPTER FOUR

THE BUILDING BLOCKS OF THE RITUAL

This chapter is all about the work of others. It is about flagging up the scientific research that should make us all think differently about what is good for us and about how we live our lives.

Two years ago I did not think about the benefits of travelling within myself. I had no idea that health could be improved and vitality and optimism accessed by closing myself within my consciousness, stilling my thoughts and bringing my focus to centre upon the body I possessed.

After days of performance of my Ritual I was aware, I think for the very first time in my life, of my inner being. I was connected to my physicality. I could visualise what was happening on the inside of my body rather than observing myself from the outside.

I paid attention to the work of the veins and muscle and bone of myself. It was as if after decades of living I became aware of the marvel of the processes that kept me alive. I can still sense the first overwhelming surge of gratitude that the initial performances of my Ritual brought. I was grateful. That is how I sum it up. I was thankful for the body that I had and I wanted to communicate my gratefulness. It was the most unusual and unlikely sensation, as if I was thanking myself, for myself and for the job every part of me was doing to sustain me.

I heard myself expressing my thanks, through affirmations, to the body I possessed and it felt good, not strange, but appropriate. I felt entirely relaxed as I allowed the sensation of gratitude to fall on every part of my body and I felt content.

Now it is a matter of course. Each and every day I communicate with my inner self, with the parts that make up the being that I am. I praise my liver, my kidneys, the cartilage that protects my joints, the blood vessels that run along my arm from my wrist to my elbow and those that run beyond. I am aware of and grateful for the work of every bodily system, response, organ, fibre, muscle and nerve ending. I recognise, at this shamefully late juncture in my life, the wonder of my engineering.

I consider my health with new optimism knowing that I need never be ill from debilitating disease. I hold with conviction the belief that disease is an invader that can be repelled by the chemistry of my body and I know as if it is a certain fact of my life, I can, through my own efforts, keep myself well.

I now connect with my body and indeed my mind in an entirely different way. It is as if my Ritual has altered the frequency to which I tune my life. I realise, compared to the manner in which I lived prior to commencing my Ritual, I now live in a different way. I find in my life circumstances unlimited possibility. I sense a potential for growth and development I have never experienced. I no longer consider age; ageing is a concept that has become irrelevant.

Within this chapter I document the four mind-body self-healing techniques I constructed my Ritual around. I did not invent them but I did combine them into a therapeutic regime

I am proud of and wish to share with others because I believe in the benefits, the Ritual as developed, can deliver. I believe it can be of as much benefit to others as to myself, reshaping other lives as it has reshaped mine.

Prior to creation of the Ritual I had read of and received anecdotal testimonies to persuade me of the possibility, and the power, each of the alternative disciplines I eventually submitted my body to, possessed, but I had never committed myself to them.

The techniques I now rely upon to empower my life are affirmation, visualisation, meditation and therapeutic touch.

Each technique is beneficial in itself. The effect of the quadrant of therapies combined is immense.

My own experience persuades me that measuring the consequences of complementary and alternative therapies is complicated. I could not now perform my Ritual without incorporating the therapeutic touch I describe in Chapter 6 and yet prior to commencement of my Ritual I had gained no benefit at all from therapies such as Reiki.

The present success of my Ritual stems I believe from the complementary power of the separate disciplines working synergistically. The results for my health and wellbeing have been extraordinary to the point that I have no doubt in stating that the four therapies when combined have an exponentially greater impact upon body and mind than that witnessed when each of the therapies was performed separately, on separate days, at different times during my week.

The hybrid-technique I created, in creating my Ritual, I perform every day by following the same pattern of movements day in and day out. I begin the series of exercises which make up my Ritual by working on my lymph system to aid lymphatic drainage,- I will show you why. I then apply my Ritual to my entire body to maintain and restore full body, physical and psychological well-being.

My aim, at the time of creation of my Ritual was to live a fuller life. A life that allowed me to reframe how I saw the potential I had within me and the future that I could create. My aim now is to do the same for you, the reader, who has chosen to buy this book.

My Ritual was not shaped over night. Initially I did not think of creating a Ritual that existed as a therapeutic tool, I just wished to pay attention to my health.

I was, as I have explained, disillusioned with my experience of mainstream medicine and reading works such as *Big Pharma* (1) made me cynical of the motivation behind billion dollar sales of pharmaceuticals. This combined with my learning about the power of placebo obviously turned my thoughts away from conventional healing techniques to … well to something of a void because I did not know what alterative route to mental and physical health to take.

What could avoid a visit to my GP, to the ten- minute state provided assessment?

(If anyone is able to tell me, what any one is able to properly assess and make decisions upon within ten minutes of following a 'flow chart' consultation? – I shall be pleased to learn!)

And let me reassure any one who thinks they may be interested to try my Ritual. I had not spent decades approaching life holistically. I had experimented with meditation as I say, affirmations, visualisation but I had not spent years of my life with alternative healers or professed myself, 'spiritually inclined'. Before performing my Ritual over and over again I could not begin to descend in to a meditative state. So take heart all of you would be novitiates for meditation is for me now an entirely natural action.

At the beginning of my quest for a health giving therapeutic regime I did what I think any sensible man would have done, I tried what had been tested and seen to deliver results. I began to incorporate, said to be effective, mind-body techniques in to my life, (out of curiosity as much as anything else), to see what any one of half a dozen different therapies could deliver. Some fell by the wayside, crystal healing I recall I could not connect with in any meaningful way. Reiki did not seem to work. I did not feel any heat or observe my purple chakra glow and flood my mind with purple light as others described. I did witness the truly astounding results Reiki delivered to others but Reiki did not work for me that is all I am able to say.

I think everyone should note that and understand with alternative healing techniques, just as with pharmaceutical remedies, the results are not the same for everyone.

THEY ONLY WORK IF YOU BELIEVE IN THEM

Not everyone responds in the same way to an anti-depressant medication, but lack of response in a section of the population does not mean the drug is withdrawn, that it is no longer NICE approved or failing to deliver benefits, to millions of others, WHO BELIEVE IN IT.

So do not quit the Ritual the day that you begin it. Quit it after a few weeks certainly if you cannot say within that time you have gained one thing from your daily performance. But make an honest assessment, even if the results obtained do not seem dramatic or startling, can you really say to yourself, you are not calmer, more positive, more focused? Even if you notice no immediate lustre in your hair or glow from your skin, consider the position honestly, do you not feel well?

If you can report no benefit at all I have to concede, as I did with crystal healing and Reiki, you are probably wasting your time. I urge you however to look elsewhere.

If you do one thing over the rest of your lifetime begin your own personal journey within to encounter the being that you are.

Over 30 years ago an Aussie doorman, on the door of a night club I was trying to get in to, told me as he waved me through, 'all we need is inside us'. He placed his finger on my chest and pressed it in as if driving the point home. He then gave me a broad smile and turned away to tap the chest of the next person in the queue. He was not, 'new age' by any stretch of the imagination, he was not drunk or high on cocaine, he was after all managing a night- club queue. He was relatively slight for a doorman with bright reddish gold hair and a freckled skin. It is his unusualness that remains with me, and the fact he was called, ' Rooney'. He seemed Irish but was Aussie through and through. He worked the door of the club for a couple of years and every time I went in I heard him tell someone, never again me. ' All we need is inside us'. The words stuck with me but I swear until I had practiced my Ritual for a prolonged period I never understood the phrase. I do now.

Turning my gaze within myself has changed, beyond any measure, I could have forseen, my exterior life. The life I construct and live with my body and my brain.

I would urge anyone to begin their own quest to find a therapeutic discipline that works to alter their own life. Changing our external perspective to a Ritual of planned inner meditation, is, I believe, where healing begins.

So let us return to my initial bumbling quest.

I had retired. I had my day to plan. I wanted to find the solution to enhancement and preservation of my health without recourse to the vast store cupboard and the millions of pills waiting for me on the shelves of twenty first century medicine. What did I do?

I set time aside to meditate. I allocated quiet time to listen to my mindfulness CD and create a meditative state. I booked therapeutic lymphatic drainage massages. In between appointments I discussed alternative therapies with my friends, asked for their assessment of the benefits. I made appointments for hopi ear candles to be placed in my ears and for hot stones to be placed along my spine. I went only once to a chant circle and not at all to river dowsing for the soul!

I engaged with open - minded people, travelled to healing centres. It all took time and effort and planning and dedication. My regime was supposed to be ancilliary to my life. I wanted it to set me up for all the adventures I had in mind, the trips I wanted to make, the hours of garden design and the coastal walks and the kite surfing leaps. Instead I was organizing my days around my journey within.

That was my grievance, but my delight was this, one very good thing occurred. I began to feel like a much younger man!

I was less tired, felt more exuberant. Certainly did not look like a man who had just retired.

I believe all readers of this book will discover that the very act of engagement with the state of their life, the state their body is in, will deliver psychological results. It is as if the very act of paying attention is enough to create optimism in the mind that the body responds to. The further act of buying a relevant book is significant enough to confirm to the mind that a quest for health has begun, which for reasons we should all now begin to understand, is an important message for the brain to receive, with important consequences for mind-body communication and physical and mental health.

I felt good and psychologically I felt empowered. There is no other word for it. I felt capable of almost anything. As capable as I did when I was 25, with as much enthusiasm and as much desire to search out new experiences.

I started making even bolder travel and leisure plans than I would have ever previously considered. I decided to take up art again.

That happened without prompting, one sunny afternoon. I dug out a random collection of old paint tubes, an easel and an already painted picture. Using the reverse side of this I painted the scene in front of my house. Carefree images flowed out of me, a painting full of blousy hydrangeas and cosmos in vibrant blues and scarlets. What next?

I looked around my home and decided to extend it. Why not? This was the attitude I had. Why not put to seemingly good use the boundless energy I had acquired?

I, you will notice, liked the consequences journeying within myself and communing with my mind, delivered to my life. I liked my regime as it was but I wanted it packaged differently.

Taking the initial steps on the journey within is a magnificent investment in oneself. I had however to concede that my regime was piecemeal and overwhelming. It took a good deal of commitment to ensure my selected range of therapies were continually included within my day.

I considered paring down my practice to focus on one thing or another, but then I had a better idea. I decided to create a therapeutic Ritual which combined aspects of all of the therapeutic approaches I had found of most benefit to me.

It is worth stating again that each technique has therapeutic merit. If you read this book and do not decide to follow my own regime I would suggest nevertheless every one incorporates at least one of the self fulfillment routines I describe within their own daily life.

Any one of the described techniques will bring about change. Each one is dynamic in its potential to trigger consequences, not only for your physical health, but also for the state of your mind and the attitude you have to life. Each method, whether it be affirmation, visualisation, meditation or therapeutic touch, will enhance the being that you are and the manner in which you experience, 'you'.

Your first performance of the Ritual may be the first time in your life you communicate with yourself. The experience

I do not doubt for those who have never believed in or tried alternative and complementary therapies will be daunting but it will also be extraordinary.

If I wrote AMAZED in seven - foot high capital letters or AWESOME on every page of this book it would not begin to capture my own reaction to the effect combining the therapies has had. By combining four of the most powerful therapeutic techniques that exist, I have not simply felt better, looked at my retirement in a different way, or radically altered my approach to maintaining my health, no, each has occurred, but the final consequence the Ritual has delivered is so, so much, more

I HAVE BEEN RENEWED

and it is this that I want for you, the reader of my book.

So let's look at the disciplines I believe in and examine the power each possesses.

AFFIRMATIONS

When we affirm something, we believe it to be true. As we say the words, affirming the facts, we know the facts stated to be the truth, and the brain records that, and that record is put to powerful effect.

Let me explain why affirmations are so important to the Ritual as it now is.

It must be clear to my readers that at the time I created my Ritual I was a man searching for something. Perhaps it happens to all of us when we reach the age of sixty.

I was in reflective and pensive mood concerning my retirement and my future when I went on a day trip to Lincoln. There, in a book – shop, I found a small book which I leafed through without any prior consideration of the force of mind-body communication or the relevance of my mind, and the thoughts I place within it, to the state of my health. Like an iconic document provided to one on a quest there existed for me this small and wondrous book, placed sideways on top of a pile of books by another browser who did not even find sufficient of interest within it to re-insert it vertically in the position from which it had been taken. It was by any assessment, 'battered', the cover torn, the waxy binding stained, and every page well thumbed with several corners creased back. It was a book that would not interest any collector wishing to buy second hand books in good condition. A book apparently read a thousand times, recently discarded and in French.

This old text that was to deliver a powerful insight in to what my Ritual should include was at that point entirely inaccessible to me through my inadequacy of language. Its message, which provides one of the fundamental building blocks of my Ritual did not enter my life until I saw the book again and I acquired a translation of the text in a book-shop in London.

Self Mastery Through Conscious Autosuggestion was the title of my small find, a book written by a French psychologist Émile Coué in 1922.

Émile Coué was a glorious and wise French man, a man of science, a pharmacist; a man who believed in the power of potions and pills. But Émile Coué was not hide bound by the doctrines of bio - chemistry, he thought in an innovative way about the power pharmaceuticals had. In delivering pills to his patients he would attach a note to describe for the patient the effectiveness of the remedy prescribed. Monsieur Coué noticed the efficacy of the drug given was enhanced when a patient had been told the drug they were to take would certainly work.

Coué believed auto-suggestion, the persuasion of the mind by the self, had an effect upon the results a drug produced. He understood the power of the mind and the role the mind has to play in healing. He was, by any sensible assessment, the forerunner of all the great scientists working today at Harvard and other great institutions to decode the power of placebo. The proponent of ideas one hundred years, at least, ahead of the time in which he lived, he is still today lauded for his insight, and indeed has been baptized, the 'Father of placebo'.

Reading this page may be the first time you have ever heard of Émile Coué. You may suggest his ideas were never tested, or that he was proposing nothing more than hypnotism.

You may balk at the idea a psychologist from a previous century may have something of vital importance to add to your life, well consider this. Émile Coué lived at the time of Einstein. Einstein's theories still form the basis of modern physics and tell us more about the Universe than any one else has discovered since. Einstein and Coué lived over 400 years after Newton published his, '*Theory of Gravitation*'. Gravity has not changed! Which allows me to suggest some ideas never go out of date, it is impossible, because they present fundamental truths that allow us to understand the world in which we exist. I suggest Émile Coué was ahead of his time. He recognised the fundamental truth that I consider will be valid for all time, that is, that the health we possess is held in our mind.

To Émile Coué a patient's mental state, that is what the patient believed, what they held in their conscious and sub-conscious mind as they swallowed a pill, affected the performance of their medication. Coué had no doubt that a particular mental state could amplify or reduce the power of the medication taken. By consciously using auto-suggestion Coué observed that his patients could cure themselves, effectively by replacing the belief that they were ill with the belief that they could be cured.

I am persuaded by his book. I have read it (my English translation) at least a dozen times. Assimilating the message it delivers is like meeting a sage in a wood who is concerned to share a secret so powerful, so fantastical, you know it has the power within it to change every other successive day for the rest of life.

Listen to this from Monsieur Coué's introduction:

(...) autosuggestion is an instrument that we possess at birth, and in this instrument, or rather in this force, resides a marvelous and incalculable power....

Monsieur Coué was of the firm belief that we possess two selves within us, our conscious and unconscious being. He believed the conscious self often demonstrates an unreliable ability to remember while the unconscious self registers the smallest, least important events of our existence and then presents them to us as an influence upon the manner in which we think and act.

In his explanation of the conscious and unconscious self within Chapter 1 of his book Émile Coué states;

(The unconscious self..., it is credulous and accepts with unreasoning docility, what it is told. Thus, as it is the unconscious that is responsible for the functioning of all our organs via the intermediary of the brain, a result is produced which may seem rather paradoxical to you: that is, if it believes that a certain organ functions well or ill, or that we feel such and such an impression, the organ in question does indeed function well or ill, or we do feel that impression. Not only does the unconscious self preside over the functions of our organism, but also over all our actions whatever they are'.

IS THAT NOT ONE OF THE MOST ASTOUNDING PROPOSITIONS YOU HAVE EVER READ?

Consider how the words of Monsieur Couè can be interpreted.

We can, if he is correct, feel, do, act, become, achieve, improve, heal, anything we want to in ourselves as long as we feed the right suggestion to our sub - conscious mind because our sub-conscious mind is suggestible and malleable and prone to believing what is fed in to it.

HOLD THIS PAGE

DO NOT TURN OVER

IF YOU TURN OVER NOW, WITHOUT UNDERSTANDING THE POINT OF WHAT YOU HAVE READ YOU WILL HAVE MISSED THE POINT OF THIS ENTIRE BOOK.

Let me take you through it again.

Auto-suggestion, that is your own message to your mind about the likely effectiveness of a drug, a surgical procedure, a healing technique, a ritual, any ritual, THE RITUAL, MY RITUAL, the one I describe in Chapter 5, will influence the result a performance of the Ritual has.

Consider all that you have learned from the opening chapters of this book. Consider what you now know about the power of belief, and imagine with wonder, what a renown psychologist born in the 19th century, admired and feted for his work in the 20th century, set down in a small book in bold type, more than 90 years ago.

Aren't you annoyed no one has told you about it before? Aren't you supremely irritated it was not on the syllabus at school? If you are reading this book as you commence or settle in to retirement, aren't you enraged that you have had to wait until what will be the final quadrant of your life to discover that in 19th century France a French man lived who was obtaining real and lasting results for his patients by changing the thoughts that they held, by filling the sub conscious mind of the ill with news that they were well?

If what Monsieur Couè taught within his lifetime is correct we can create not only the state of health we wish for, but the life we wish for, driven by the capabilities we announce to our sub-conscious mind that we possess.

We must not engage our will. Monsieur Coué was very firm about that. It is our unconscious self we must persuade by repeated auto- suggestion as to the out come desired. Monsieur Coué argued that we cannot cure an alcoholic by asking his will to perform differently by refusing a drink. Alcoholics drink, criminals commit crime, because an alcoholic and a thief imagine they cannot prevent themselves from drinking, stealing, committing acts of burglary. Imagination is the unconscious self; it is what is in the imagination that must be changed. If the imagination is changed successfully the will of an individual can be directed. In the words of Monsieur Coué

'Thus, we, who are so proud of our will, who believe we are free to act as we like, are in reality nothing but wretched puppets of which our imagination holds all the strings. We have only ceased to be puppets when we have learned to guide our imagination.'

Taming the imagination is in Coué's terms like putting a bridle on a horse.

In Coué's theory there is no division between our imagination and our unconscious self. The unconscious being is the imaginative being and the imagination can be programmed, altered, benefited by auto -suggestion. Auto-suggestion is the acceptance by the patient's subconscious of a statement made by another, (a therapist or a hypnotist) or the acceptance by the sub conscious of a statement the patient makes to him or herself.

Acceptance of the statement made, as a result of my exhortation to myself in the steam of my bathroom mirror!

ACCEPTANCE!

Let us stop there.

Do you get it?

CYNICS PUT THIS BOOK DOWN.

THROW IT AWAY.

IT IS OF ABSOLUTELY NO USE TO YOU.

IT CAN SERVE ABSOLUTELY NO PURPOSE IN YOUR LIFE.

If you are staying with me, and continuing to read what I write, you must be prepared to believe in what I tell you now and Monsieur Coué told his patients over ninety years ago.

WE CAN TELL OURSELVES WHAT TO THINK, WHAT TO BELIEVE, AND OUR STATEMENTS CAN EFFECT HOW WE ARE, HOW WE LIVE, HOW WE AGE, HOW WE HEAL, HOW WE BEHAVE, HOW WE EXIST

We can persuade our inner self that AWESOME is our reality, that our potential, as the human being we are born, is unlimited.

We are limited by only one thing, THE LIMIT WE PLACE UPON OUR SELF, the information we place in our unconscious self, that is, our imagination.

We can just as easily brainwash ourselves to believe that a daily therapeutic Ritual is doing us good, is making our organs function, our skeleton strong, our sinews flexible, our minds alert and our body agile as we can think negatively and persuade our unconscious, that the self that we are is unlikely to achieve anything in our lives, that we are held captive by circumstances, prone to disease, likely as time progresses to decay and decline until decrepid we reach our death.

Is it a type of brainwashing?

OF COURSE IT IS A TYPE OF BRAINWASHING

I know BRAINWASHING is a term with many negative connotations. The meaning behind the word most easily summed up by the villain in a psychological thriller or the dictator controlling the minds of his people, but brainwashing in itself is not negative. It depends on the facts we are feeding in to our mind and the motivation behind the exercise that determines what we are trying to achieve.

Èmile Coué did not brainwash his patients, in negative terms, neither did he put them to sleep to hypnotise them. Instead Monsieur Coué reached the sub-conscious mind of a patient by repeating to the patient in slow monotonous and soothing rhythm the beneficial and restorative facts Monsieur Coué wished the sub-conscious to accept as deep and profound truth.

Monsieur Coué worked with his patients in this way and then he allowed them to take over for themselves.

In 1922 Coué believed in the power of autosuggestion so strongly, in its beneficial potential for the healing process, he set down in his book that:

'(...) I should like to see the theoretical and practical study of suggestion on the syllabus of the medical schools for the great benefit of the sick and of the doctors themselves....'

Has your Doctor ever mentioned it?

Mine certainly has not; such a positive and beneficial aspect of preservation, maintenance and enhancement of ourselves, not once incorporated in to any consultation with any medical practitioner I have taken part in, in my life.

What a marvellous and ingenious gift built in to every human being. Like a booster set of rockets or additional gear levers never accessed.

Astounding, incomprehensible, beyond belief! UNTIL YOU TRY IT FOR YOURSELF.

Coué, clearly believed it was a huge leap for the average man or woman living in 1922 to accept that autosuggestion, the statements communicated to their unconscious self by their conscious self, could, a) really have a dramatic effect on health, perception, condition, behaviour and b) be a tool the patient could apply upon themselves without the need for intervention of or payment to a therapist.

To persuade those living in his time to accept the concept he created a sequence of practical demonstrations to educate patients as to the power contained within the sub-conscious mind.

I pause briefly at this point to honour Monsieur Coué's persistence in endeavouring to communicate his message. If this intelligent, forward thinking man, was alive to the unlikeliness of acceptance of his glittering proposition in 1922, what would he think of those who would rail against his technique and positively decry it in 2014? Certainly more vehemently with more scientific data clenched within their fists than Monsieur Coué had probably ever seen.

Our world has advanced. We have clean water, immunisation against disease, laser surgery, silicon chips, but our minds have closed. Rationality is the victor now, our imaginations are locked within themselves, but they are not removed. We each possess the gift of belief, of creative thought. Our power to imagine has not been taken, it has simply been sidelined as a therapeutic tool. Who did that? Why were people made well in 1922 by turning within themselves and in 2014 we consider it some kind of voodoo? Well, although it is disappointing to express this, it is my opinion that vested interests and the structures within modern medicine prevent the promotion of any technique that is not acceptable to those who manage resources or have power. If they don't like it, we can't have it. Well not unless we access it for ourselves.

These are the messages I send to myself, to my sub-conscious mind, as my Ritual begins.

I AM AWESOME

THE BEST IN MY LIFE IS AHEAD OF ME

I AM DISEASE FREE

I AM AS FIT AS I WAS AT 28

Monsieur Coué's quietly spoken mantras, his elegant suit and watch chain, his fixed stare in to his patient's eye and commands delivered were all part, I believe, of Monsieur

Coué's ritual to instill belief, in the mind of the patient, in the facts Monsieur Couè pronounced. Monsieur Coué did more than provide his patients with a list of affirmations to repeat, he created for each patient their own personal ritual to bring about desired change.

I was slowly recognising that to unleash the power we have within us, to shape and redefine our life and our health, a ritual of some kind is required. A ritual is I believe the scaffold the unconscious self pulls its self up upon to direct our body to respond to the information the sub-conscious provides.

Monsieur Coué was not modest in describing the benefits of his technique of auto-suggestion. Coué' proposed his technique had the power within it to cure illness and he did not propose that tentatively. He was very definite about the responsibility each individual has for their own health and for maintenance and preservation of the body they have been given. Coué believed we have the power within us to keep ourselves well and he boldly stated this in his book.

"Before sending away your patient you must tell him that he carries within him the instrument by which he can cure himself, and that you are, as it were, only a professor teaching to use the instrument"

And with even more boldness and enthusiasm:

" After what has just been said it would seem that nobody ought to be ill. That is quite true. Every illness, whatever it may be, can yield to autosuggestion, daring and unlikely as my statement may seem; I do not say does always yield, but can yield, which is a different thing"

I read his short book a dozen times before I created the Ritual. I wove his principles in to my daily programme and do you know what? After several years of my Ritual performance I agree with him.

Perform my Ritual, (or your variation of it), once a day for six weeks. Or if you will not do that, so that I know I am not in your debt, do only what Monsieur Coué' advises. Lie on your bed or look at yourself in the mirror and affirm, because it is a fact.

I AM A MAGNIFICENT UNLIMITED BEING WITH THE POTENTIAL WITHIN ME TO ACHIEVE ANYTHING I WISH TO ACHIEVE

THERAPEUTIC TOUCH

Touch is good for us.

Touch directs our mind to heal the body we possess.

Both statements are true but you will never benefit from the power of therapeutic touch without recognising something fundamental about yourself.

You are not just flesh and blood and viscera and bone. That is only one way of looking at the situation. To open your mind to the gift of therapeutic touch and the impact it can have upon illness, existence, day to day living, you have to see yourself from another angle. You are not just matter. Indeed, you may not know it, but there is a war going on in science. A war of words to decide, if we are matter, (the perspective you may like to hang on to, the sit on the sofa, flesh and bloodness of us all,) or we are energy. What is inside our cells, what are our atoms made of? – matter and density or energy and light?

We are not just blood and guts and organs and skeletal frame. Those descriptors don't begin to go far enough. To recognise what a human being is we have to remember it depends upon who is asking the question. A physicist, plumping for matter or energy; a biologist, plumping for the blood and guts of our cellular structure or a chemist, announcing, 99% of what we are is made up of six elements, oxygen, carbon, hydrogen, nitrogen, calcium and phosphorus. We are in fact according to our chemistry, more than 50% water.

So when I try to tell you about life energy and the mechanism of therapeutic touch, the means practitioners believe by which energy can be harnessed balanced and directed, do not slam this book shut. (Not for the umpteenth time!) I know it is challenging. I know you like the truths within your life, which are familiar, to be protected and maintained. I understand you have been content with the 10 minute GP appointment and content to take the prescription drugs delivered with your name upon the sachet or the box, but I am not prepared to allow you that life in tact. I want you to recognise your life, the life you actually possess, is far more complicated than that.

If this is the first time in your life you have been confronted with the reality that bio –chemical medicine may not be the fix all you need, hallelujah, because the future is opening up to you.

You have within you the energy of life drawn from a source much greater than yourself. You carry it. It is not extinguished until your life is ended and in the meantime it is yours to draw upon to re-energise, restore and bless your life, and in its application, heal yourself if you are ill, renew yourself if you are fatigued or re-energise yourself if you are only disconnected or depressed.

Every faith in the world recognises the energy I am talking about. To Christians it is made manifest by miracles, by the biblical 'laying on of hands' through the work of the Virgin Mary and of Christ. To Chinese culture it is ch'i or qi. To Hindu culture it is prana. To Hawaiian culture, 'mana'. In Tibetan Buddhism it is lüng.

Our connection to a force much greater than the sum power of all of our cells is what energy practitioners and healers from around the world, in a myriad of different expressions, stemming from a global quantity of different cultures work with and it is this energy that makes powerful therapeutic touch.

Is all touch therapeutic?

Is there a difference between the touch you can apply to yourself, with your own hands and the touch a healer applies? Having subjected myself to the Ritual and witnessed the benefits I don't think so, and by the time you get to the end of this section it may be that you agree with me.

What do you do when you walk in to the corner of a coffee table and hit the centre of your knee so hard against it you expect to see shards of bone lying on the ground?

Well, depending upon who you are, I imagine you jump around railing in suppressed exhortation against everything in the world or you openly curse.

Our reactions differ; our responses are dictated by our upbringing, by what we consider acceptable words to use. We determine through our history what constitutes a decent level of outburst, but every one of us, regardless of the source of instruction that guides us, regardless of race or where we hail from, does this: we hold ourselves tightly, and then rub, and rub again and again at the site of the injury while pressing our palm firmly in to our skin.

Why do we do that?

And why do we do it instinctively from the time we are a child; from the time memory begins and possibly even before we know we store memory, and why do we do it every time injury strikes us?

Because it takes the pain away, isn't that the answer?

HOW DOES TOUCH DO THAT?

Why does touch have such power within it and why is the result of touch the same for every being living on this planet?

Biologically something happens.

Ever noticed that? The increasing redness at the site we draw our brain's attention to. The sudden heat of our blood directed to the site of our injury.

There are longer - term consequences. Bruising is less if an injured part of the body is rubbed and massaged after a blow is suffered, but what is it that happens in our brain when touch is applied?

Is the brain distracted or directed?

I used to think the former and now I am most definite it is the latter.

In placebo experiments patients have been made to concentrate on sending blood in to their hands and when measurements have been taken by the scientists involved the concentration of blood in the fingers and palms of patients has increased. A dummy placebo pill has even been shown to have the power to impact upon the manner in which blood circulates and to reduce systolic blood pressure. Of course it was not the pill, because the pill was inert, it was the mind, directed by the patient's belief, that a pill had been given which had the power to impact upon blood pressure. The mind altered the pressure a patient's blood registered. (2)

The evident way in which we direct our mind to increase blood flow at the site of a 'knock' or 'blow', convinces me we have the means within us to direct our mind to the task of minimizing the consequences of an injury. Our touch is I believe the signal that calls on the brain to marshall the resources within us to send our blood to the site at which it is needed. If the brain can do that for as insignificant a matter as a blow against a coffee table edge, is it not likely the brain will wish to engage itself in circumstances of a full on assault upon our being?

As I performed my Ritual I considered this question. I asked myself, are my channels of communication between my body and my brain opened only in the event of injury or assault or can the application of touch engage my brain to orchestrate my body to respond, not to deliver respite and healing after injury, but to tackle or prevent degeneration and decay? Can therapeutic touch rally the arsenal of the mind to the task of body maintenance or even to the more complicated labour of regeneration?

Massage of any kind is good for us we know that. A therapist delivered massage stimulates pressure receptors under the skin, which increases nerve activity in the brain. This has been demonstrated to lead to an increase in levels of serotonin within the brain, and a reduction in levels of the stress hormone cortisol. High cortisol levels are known to challenge the body's defences and weaken the immune system leaving us more open to disease.

The Cincinnati Children's Hospital uses healing touch therapy to stimulate wound healing, and provide pain relief. Trials at Stanford University in the US have demonstrated that touch therapy does accelerate wound healing, relieves pain and anxiety and may have positive effects on a variety of orthopaedic conditions, including healing fractures and healing muscle and connective tissue.(3)

Before I began to write the Ritual I did not appreciate the extent of research carried out in to the benefits of therapeutic touch. I certainly had no idea that the University of Miami had invested in its very own Touch Research Institute dedicated to studying the effects of touch therapy.

The institute at Miami has conducted over 100 studies dedicated to understanding the therapeutic consequences of massage. Research findings demonstrate that massage triggers some astounding consequences.

Premature infants develop more rapidly if massaged, compared to infants from whom massage is withheld; patients suffering from fibromyalgia experience less pain : asthmatics breathe more easily and demonstrate greater lung function; the glucose levels of patients with diabetes falls following massage. One of the most remarkable testimonies to the power of massage is that those subjecting themselves to a massage regime, have, according to the Touch Research Institute's website, a greater number of 'killer- cells' present within the body as compared to those who never experience massage. This has consequences for the long -term health of patients suffering diseases such as HIV and cancer.

WHY DOES NO ONE TELL US THESE THINGS!

And what about touching ourselves? Can self - applied massage deliver beneficial effects?

Is my Ritual effective because I deliver to myself all of the benefits scientists have recorded from massage delivered by therapists?

I believe so.

I firmly believe by incorporating touch within my Ritual massage I enhance communication between my body and my mind. I, if you like, direct my mind to engage and conduct its healing performance as I move my hands around my body.

And I am not sick. I am not calling the attention of my mind to injury but to a daily overhaul of the being that I am. Whole body maintenance is achieved I believe when the mind is led by touch and massage to engage.

Am I self- healing? - or self –maintaining? - or, engaging in a type of self –restoration? I certainly feel younger and in a better state of health than I did when my Ritual began?

Can therapeutic touch work just as effectively if it is self-applied without a doctor, therapist or shaman intervening and can current science answer that question?

At this point in the early 21st Century I am afraid science cannot fully answer my question but ongoing research at University College London inspires me to believe I am on the right path.

In 2010 a team of scientists from the Institute of Cognitive Neuroscience at University College London led by Professor Patrick Haggard and Marjolein Kammers demonstrated self-touch has the ability to reduce a sensation of acute pain by up to 64%. The experiment constructed used the thermal grill illusion to assess the pain relief patients gained in an injured index finger when the finger was pressed against fingers of the other hand.

The thermal grill illusion has been used in scientific experiment from the 19th century onwards. It is created when two hot objects are placed around a cool object. Touching the unbearably hot objects first, prior to touching the cool object, causes the cool object to also deliver a sensation of unbearable heat. In the UCL experiment the index and ring fingers of trial participants were placed in hot water and the middle finger in cold water. The consequence was a sensation of heat in the middle finger. To alleviate this pain participants were allowed to press the fingers of their two hands together. Greater pain relief was delivered when three fingers of each hand were engaged and pressed against each other. Pain in the middle finger fell by 64%. If only one or two fingers were pressed together less pain relief was experienced and pain relief was also less *if participants pressed their painful middle finger against another's hand instead of against their own.*

Self- touch reduced pain considerably more than any pain relief provided through touch from others.

The work of the team at University College London persuades me that the mind and body have a method of working together to respond to injury which is self - supporting and as powerful, if not more effective, as the solution delivered when a therapist intervenes.

My belief in therapeutic touch explains why my Ritual is constructed in the way that it is. Each exercise in the Ritual whether for body or face, whether for maintenance, restoration, or re-sculpting of my tissues through work in the 'recumbent gym', begins with positioning the finger- tips on the area of skin to be worked upon.

The state I create within myself when my Ritual is performed, is one I describe as 'overwhelming awareness of the physicality of me'. It is akin to full body mindfulness.

Mindfulness is the form of meditation that is 'all the rage' at the moment. Indeed I am moved by the sudden overwhelming popularity of this discipline, as if mindfulness is an alpha state that has only just been invented, when in fact mindful- meditation has been an essential part of Buddhist and Hindu culture for over 2500 years.

It is as if all of us, not just myself, are searching in this century of riches, for a route to living fully, and it may be that we are all beginning to understand the things most required within our lives are not found in the app store but in history and wisdom refined over thousands of years.

The difference between mindful meditation and the meditative act of my Ritual is that the Ritual is, as a result of the incorporation of therapeutic touch, mindfulness directed. The alpha state created is not simply experienced but directed to the task of restoration of life energy and renewal of the body and the brain.

MEDITATION

It's all the rage. Wherever you look there are posters for free meditation sessions. Fashion magazines, articles on current affairs, sell out books on how to be successful in business, all tell you the same thing; if you want to succeed you have to do things mindfully.

Mindfulness is the new mantra of those with time on their hands.

It is important, as I have said, to remind ourselves, that mindfulness meditation was not invented in the 21st century, even though our recent enthusiasm for the art suggests it is our own sparkling new method of paying attention.

It is almost as if mindfulness was created in 2010, it only being in the last handful of years, that growing numbers of us have snatched at the concept in the hope of garnering its power for ourselves.

We are aware meditation comes from the East. We know it has something to do with Buddhists and for the majority of us that is the limit of our understanding. Save we know, 'we have never done it', mindfully or otherwise. The majority of us have never meditated.

And here we should address the inter -changeability with which we all discuss mindfulness and meditation. Mindfulness is not the same as an act of meditation. Mindfulness is a means of processing the information our brain receives and the thoughts we create. Mindfulness does not require us to sit still, close our eyes and listen to a tape of the rain forest. Mindfulness is a way of life and when perfected can turn our act of living in to an art.

When we are mindful we pay attention. We live entirely in the moment with our perspective unclouded by past reality or the prospect of future events unfolding in a particular way. We connect with the actions we perform without imposing our judgment.

Mindful meditation is the tool we can use to help us to lead a mindful life in which every action is performed mindfully. When we meditate mindfully we are aware of our thoughts. Our motivation is not to eliminate thought and create a blank screen; our motivation is instead to be aware of our thoughts and to recognise we exist apart from them. Thoughts form and dissipate and form again. Thoughts are representative of the activity in our mind, of our cognitive processing, but they are only thoughts.

We are more than the thoughts we possess.

Once this is realised we are empowered to alter our perspective, creating different emotional responses in our life to the thoughts that we carry.

Cognitive behavioural therapists use mindful meditation techniques as a tool of therapy to enable emotion to be disassociated from particular thought patterns so placing patients back in control of their life. Adverts advertising the benefit of mindfulness based cognitive therapy are suddenly everywhere. Mindfulness therapy promises the end of addiction, of life freed from destructive patterns of behavior, from the over load of stressful living.

Wow! No wonder we are all so keen to live mindfully.

But don't lose sight of the fact that mindfulness is only one approach to journeying within.

I was alive in the 1960's. If I had not created and subjected myself to my Ritual I would say that the 1960's represented the 'decade' of my life. But since I have been ' Ritualising', I await with similar anticipation 2020. Nevertheless I recall in the 1960's the popularity of transcendental meditation. The obsession the Beatles had with transcendental meditation and their trip to India in 1968 to study with Maharishi Mahesh Yogi.

The interest the Beatles had in transcendental meditation changed the attitude many westerners displayed towards meditation. The consequence of the association of celebrity with meditative practice was a huge upsurge of interest in the practice in Europe and the United States, but even that demonstrable rise in the popularity of Eastern spirituality and meditative techniques was not nearly so widespread as the present interest in mindful meditation as a tool for aiding good health.

One reason for this, I consider, is the publication of many recent scientific studies which have produced hard evidence that meditation has a beneficial impact on our brain. Indeed has the power to change the very shape our brain possesses.

The Beatles would have experienced the same benefit as those meditating today in 2014. The difference is, that today, the brain scanning techniques we possess, did not exist in the 1960's and so the Beatles even though ensuring an Eastern meditative technique made an impression on an otherwise impervious West could not carry home with them brain scans to document the real benefit for the brain, the creation of a meditative state can create.

When we meditate we induce a particular state of consciousness. The act of meditating is an act of inward contemplation that is not specific to any one religion or race. Meditation encompasses the mindful meditation of the Buddhists, the spiritual meditation of Hindus, the transcendental act that so attracted the Beatles and the kind of meditation a person can perform sitting in an armchair simply by closing their eyes and listening to a meditative CD they have acquired in a health food shop.

Meditation is the act of journeying within. When we meditate we separate our consciousness from our external worldly life. We journey inside ourselves to a place in consciousness that is not filled with our memorabilia, our cars, our three piece suites, our art collection or tracks on our I-pod; it is the vast space of our beginning. Through meditation we arrive at the unwritten hard disk of our self and stay there as long as the state of consciousness, meditation creates, prevails.

The purpose of Hindu and Buddhist religious meditation is to empower the human being to seek and attain enlightenment or align with their own divinity. The meditative act as a religious and spiritual device is the method by which the earthly ego is transcended and a greater self revealed.

In Western society meditation has been re-invented as a secular device for promotion of good health.

The Eastern spiritual technique, re-packaged by medics, psychologists and self help therapists in the US and Europe is not intended to raise us towards a celestial plane but to lower our levels of stress, diminish anxiety and strengthen our immunity against disease.

In the United States meditation is widely used in hospitals to alleviate the symptoms of patients suffering from chronic stress, chronic pain and acute anxiety. In the UK mindfulness therapy is a NICE approved therapy for recurrent depression. (4)

It is reported the Mental Health Foundation estimate that 30% of GP's now refer patients to mindfulness training. (5) Indeed if you click on the NHS website and enter 'mindfulness' you will receive a full explanation as to why mindfulness is good for you and the benefits for the health of mindful meditation.

WHY?

What explains this sudden endorsement by the NHS of mindful meditation?

I would suggest the incontrovertible evidence that mindful meditation delivers results!

MRI imaging is able to provide us with brightly coloured scans demonstrating brain activity is affected beneficially by a period of daily meditation lasting no longer than eight weeks. Vivid MRI scans document changes that occur in neural activity when meditation occurs. Studies demonstrate meditation raises immunity and reduces anxiety and stress. Moreover meditation changes the way in which the brain processes information with consequential benefits for breaking addiction and improving depression.

A study published in the Journal of Psychosomatic Medicine in 2002, entitled,

Alterations in Brain and Immune Function Produced by Mindfulness (6) concluded that a short course of mindful meditation lasting only 8 weeks can change brain and immune function in positive ways. Changed patterns of brain activity associated with positive benefits were witnessed. In the trial, trial participants required to meditate produced a greater number of anti-bodies, following injection with a flu vaccine, as compared to others within a control group who did not meditate, even though all participants in both groups had received a flu vaccination.

Your Brain On Meditation an article published in *Psychology Today,* by Rebecca Gladding M.D in February 2013 tells us in technical terms which areas of the brain are affected when we meditate and in what way. (7) The thesis of the article is that meditation alters neural pathways between different sectors of the brain changing the dominance of different areas of the brain in the processing of information. Rebecca Gladding proposes this alteration is beneficial in that it allows individuals to process information less emotively and to exhibit greater empathy and compassion towards others in their life.

Information about the scientifically documented benefits of meditation is generously made available on the internet by the Harvard Medical School, the University of Massachusetts Medical School, and the Benson Henry Institute within the Massachusetts General Hospital. Take a look at these web sites. Consider for yourself the reported benefits of meditation. I consider any reasonably intelligent man or woman able to read about the work of this group of scientists will be converted in to a habitual meditator, virtually over night.

Studies conducted by Professor Henry Benson and his colleagues at the Harvard Medical School have shown that deep meditation changes our bodies on a genetic level. Researchers identified more disease fighting genes in long - term practitioners of yoga and meditation compared to those present in subjects not practising any form of meditation. The study confirms what biologists have already established, that our genes can switch to an 'on' position from an 'off' position and vice versa. In those who meditate, genes that protect the body from cancer, fight inflammation and produce natural bodily defences, all began to switch 'on' after a programme of meditation lasting only eight weeks.

Sarah Lazar from the Harvard Medical School has documented an increase in grey matter in the brains of those who meditate. (8) After an eight week programme of meditation structural changes were seen in the cerebral cortex of study participants; the cerebral cortex thickening in areas associated with attention and emotional integration.

A further study in 2011 allowed Sarah Lazar and her colleagues to study MRI scans produced of the brains of 16 trial participants, two weeks before and two weeks after they took part in an 8 week meditation programme, within the Centre for Mindfulness, operated by the University of Massachusetts. The consequences of participating in a Mindfulness Based Stress Reduction Programme for an average of 27 minutes per day for a period of 8 weeks was a thickening of grey matter within the hippocampus, an area of the brain important for learning and memory, as well as in structures within the brain associated with compassion and introspection.

IT IS VERY IMPORTANT THAT WE APPRECIATE WHAT THESE SCIENTISTS ARE TELLING US!

The reported studies document observable clinical results and changes within the brains and conditions of patients who meditate, within a period of 8 weeks.

It is also suggested that patients who meditate have lower cortisol levels and so present as less stressed. The size of the amygdala, the area of the brain involved in responding to fear and threat is reduced, moderating flight impulses.

Elissa Epel, a psychologist at the University of California has expressed the opinion that meditation 'may boost pathways of restoration and health enhancement', 'perhaps by triggering a release of growth and sex hormones'. (9)

IMAGINE THE CONSEQUENCE FOR YOUR HEALTH OF ADOPTING SOME FORM OF MEDITATIVE

PRACTICE OR RITUAL OVER THE REST OF YOUR LIFETIME.

It need not be a programme of mindfulness meditation.

The Benson – Henry Institute offers the advice that it can be any similar programme as long as the consequence is a change in the thought patterns of the individual concerned. Diaphragmatic breathing, repetitive prayer, chi gong, tai chi, yoga, progressive muscle relaxation, jogging, even knitting are all given as examples of a meditative regime sufficient to produce results.

I suggest my Ritual.

The Ritual has a regime of meditation built in to it. Indeed the connection required between the mind and the physical body, if the Ritual is to deliver results, can only be made in a state of mindful concentration.

And do not be discouraged. It does not matter if on the first occasion you attempt to perform the Ritual your head is invaded by external noise, not only from the activities of others, but also from your own brain. Brains throw in a barrage of unhelpful thought as soon as we try to meditate. But I know from personal experience, and studies have also shown, the more we try to meditate, the more proficient we become and the more effective the meditative state produced is.

Professor of Medicine Emeritus Jon Kabat – Zinn, founder and former director of the Stress Reduction Clinic at the University of Massachusetts Medical Centre, was one of the first in the field of mind – body medicine to pronounce the benefits for the body of regular meditation. John Kabat -Zinn is recognised as a practitioner who has, through his work, probably done more than any other to integrate Eastern meditative rituals in to main - stream Western medicine. Jon Kabat - Zinn suggests the ideal regime for meditation to obtain maximum benefit from a meditative practice is a regime of 6 x 45minute sessions in any one week. (10)

My daily Ritual is not based upon this opinion, my Ritual was created before I was aware of Professor Zinn's suggestion, but the meditative period of time suggested by the Professor correlates almost exactly with the time I dedicate to my Ritual, save that my Ritual is performed over one extra day. I recommend performance of my Ritual on every day of the week. Indeed I recommend that you perform my Ritual, or your own version of it, every day for the rest of your life.

VISUALISATION

Visualisation is the last powerful therapeutic device I incorporate in to my Ritual.

It is the use of the imagination to produce vivid images in the brain to support the beneficial outcome we wish to achieve for our body or in our life.

Visualisation is not a weird new age technique, that any sensible person should want nothing to do with. It is not performed only by those who visit Glastonbury or those who turn up before sunrise or before the frost falls to witness the summer or winter solstice. No it is not that. It is a device used for thousands of years in Buddhist and Hindu traditions to restore harmony to the mind and to the body. It is respected, effective and understood to be powerful not only by practitioners in the East, but by practitioners in the West.

Not only for the impact it may have upon minor scrapes or trifling diseases, no, visualisation is not a tool limited to the cure of headaches, or stiffness in the legs, it is a 21st century NHS approved treatment method to deal with symptoms of our very modern tragedies, cancer and aids.

Ok, if this really is the time you are going to shout, 'rubbish', at the air around you and hurl my book away – don't. Take a look instead at the Cancer Research UK website and consider what it says about visualisation.

Cancer Research UK recognise visualisation as a useful technique to manage the symptoms of cancer. It is promoted as a technique capable of relieving stress and anxiety and boosting the immune system of those afflicted by cancer.

The words on the website are clear and unambiguous:

I quote:

What visualisation is:

The idea behind visualisation is that you use the power of your imagination to help relieve symptoms or manage problems. Learning to direct and control images in your mind can help you to relax. This may help to;

Relieve Stress

Control some of the symptoms caused by your cancer or cancer treatments

Boost your immune system to help your body fight off infections and promote healing.

Some of our very best UK scientists and researchers work with Cancer Research UK. I find it heartening that this website should offer those suffering from cancer an explanation of the power of visualisation and propose it as a technique, to aid an individual in their battle to confront this awful disease.

The approach taken by Cancer Research UK demonstrates a shift of perspective from doctors and scientists battling this disease, away from absolute homage to powerful pharmaceuticals to acknowledgement of the worth of therapies that have nothing at all to do with drugs and a lot to do with instilling hope. The site demonstrates a laudable open mindedness and a willingness to overlay the pharmaceutical driven regime of the West with the holistic nature of traditions from the East. It represents a 'global' approach to medicine, combining world knowledge of what it is that heals; applying the best of everything, sourced from any tradition, to stop the ravages of disease.

I urge you all who wish to live a better life, who wish to squeeze the juice from existence, to

LIVE IN YOUR TIME.

Take what is available to you. Try the manufactured drugs, have a severely broken leg pinned by the latest type of resilient and complex screw that adjusts its torque to allow your bone to heal. Why wouldn't you? But don't stop there, don't live partially in your time. Take all the knowledge that exists in this world in 2014 and apply it to your life.

That includes welcoming in other disciplines, making the unusual, the unfamiliar, part of your health regime. You have not been brought up on 'airy fairy' thinking. You have never sat still, just for the purpose of closing your eyes and creating images that may 'heal' you. You do not even recognise that 'healing' may be something more than a rash disappearing, bronchitis clearing from your chest, or back pain subsiding.

HEALING IS NOT ALL ABOUT THE SYMPTOMS YOU PRESENT.

HEALING IS REBOOTING THE COMPUTER OF YOURSELF getting rid of the bugs and viruses you may not know even exist.

If you commit yourself to the Ritual you accept you have a fourth dimension, you place yourself in a world mainstream medicine is only beginning to understand. Remember, fifty years from now, when the newly made surgeons are dead or retiring, all the techniques they were astounded by and could not wait to try out, will be outmoded, 'old hat', not something you would allow to be used on your own son or daughter or wife if you were alive in 2079.

So break out of any pattern of thinking that tells you every answer lies in the medical textbooks or with the surgeons, GP's and consultants of today. You do not have to defect to the East, but you have to let the approach and traditions of the East in to your daily life. If you are to live fully and long, in good health, you must recognise the power within yourself and your responsibility to work with the mind that you have, to deliver that self good health.

Akira Otani, from the University of Maryland Counseling Centre, in an article entitled *Eastern Meditative Techniques and Hypnosis: A New Synthesis* (11) sums up the competing strengths, merits and drawbacks of Eastern v Western healing paradigms. Essentially, she concludes, the West is best at critical intervention, the East is best at whole life wellness and at turning the body in to a vehicle, to travel through life in, avoiding the debilitation of chronic disease.

So even if you have never heard of visualisation;

GIVE IT A GO. USE IT, FOR THE BEST OF IT IS, VISUALISATION IS EASY, EFFECTIVE AND POWERFUL AND IT IS GOOD FOR YOU!

Scientists over the last couple of decades have been studying the effects of visualization and the results are remarkable.

Those who are crippled by neurological disease have found benefit in visualising improvements in motor control. (12) Motor imagery is the 'mental representation of movement without movement.' Visualising improved motor skills and performance has led to positive results in terms of increased speed in athletes, improvements in muscle strength and movement dynamics, but remarkably there is emerging evidence that visualising motor imagery can also improve motor and task performance in those with the most debilitating neurologic disease.

In 2000 scientists in North Carolina. (13) carried out a psychoneuroimmunological study to examine the effects of visualisation on the immune system response of patients suffering with AIDS. In particular the scientists wished to examine the effectiveness of AIDS patients visualising their own white cells multiplying and increasing in number. Ten male and ten female participants took part in the study, among them medical patients diagnosed with cancer, AIDS, viral infections, and other medical problems associated with a depressed white blood cell count. Results of the study indicated significant increases in white blood count in all patients over a period of 90 days.

My favourite study documenting the positive results of a programme of visualisation is that conducted by a group of scientists in Canada. (14) The study tested whether mental training alone could increase muscular strength. Thirty athletes were assigned to perform mental training of their hip flexor muscles, thirty others were assigned to use equipment in a gym to train the same muscles and thirty others within a control group did not visualise or train in a gym. Mental training increased physical strength by 24%, gym training increased muscle strength by 28%, there was no significant alteration in muscle strength among athletes in the control group.

I was so awe struck by the outcome of this study and the possibilities that visualisation presented I created a series of Ritual exercises dedicated to keeping myself in shape. The programme which, results I set out, in The Recumbent Gym. Be aware when you consider the photographic imagery the muscles in my torso and my arms have been made by my mind!

A further review of the benefits of guided visualisation conducted in 2008 confirmed visualisation can reduce stress and elevate the immune system (15)

Would you have thought it?

Really!

If I had said to you: ' come on it's winter, let's boost your immunity; relax, sit down and take yourself inside your head and once there imagine all is well, there is sunlight on the lake of your life, and look the sun is rising and it is carrying within itself, in every vibrant ray, powerful healing energy rising inside you like a beacon'. Would you have given it a go or would you have gone for your flu jab!!

I bet the way you viewed things before you picked up the Ritual you would have gone for the jab. And that's fine! That is the point of living in your time. Take all that is on offer and live the best life you can, but if you have never tried it I urge you to begin today to incorporate visualisation in to your every day life.

If you are to obtain benefits from my Ritual you must become evangelistic about your own health and future longevity. We are all capable of laziness, of buying self-help guides and keeping them on the shelf, but I am sharing with you information that can have a radical effect on your wellbeing. It is worth dedicating just a little of your time to achieve the massive benefits the Ritual will deliver. The more excited and passionate you get about your performance of the Ritual, the greater, I promise you, the benefits that will be delivered

It is important to me that my Ritual incorporates targeted visualisation of images I invent for my body. Visualisation makes the whole process of travelling within easier. Either borrow imagery from an anatomy textbook or invent your body as you wish it to be, a flower garden, a race track, a machine.

I assure you, anyone can do it. If you think visualisation is not for you, or that creating mental imagery is beyond your mental gifts, take heart. A Japanese study in 2005 (16) considered the effects of a programme of guided visualisation upon a number of healthy subjects. Results demonstrated that the longer participants practised visualising the better they became at producing vivid images within their imagination. Short term or inexperienced practitioners were less able to produce vivid visual images. The greater the period of time over which trial participants incorporated a session of visualisation in to their day, the more adept they were at creating visual imagery and the lower their stress scores became and the higher their scores on markings of their all round general health.

I think any one who has never given the act of visualisation a go should take heart from such study results. I stress that the benefits my Ritual is able to deliver will not come to you over night.

PRACTISE AND BELIEVE; PRACTISE AND BELIEVE; PRACTISE AND BELIEVE it is all that I can tell you.

THE RITUAL DOES NOT DELIVER IMMEDIATE RESULTS IT DELIVERS LASTING RESULTS THAT COME WITH PRACTISE.

It will get easier and part of that ease I believe is due to the opening of channels between the mind and the body which we never regularly use and indeed only access when we journey within. We have a fourth dimension, let's use it and let's keep it simple.

When I visualise I do not create any complicated imagery. I just cannot do it. I have been told that visualisation practitioners offering guided visualisation narrate while visualisation is ongoing offering descriptions of tranquil scenery to induce calm and assist beginners to hold an imagined scene in their brain. Cancer is often seen as a black cloud gradually pierced and dissolved by bright light until the only cloud remaining is white and the sky around it is blue.

I have heard of images being constructed of steel jawed dogs eating rabid toxic cells and wiping them out. The AIDs patients mentioned in the experiment above were required to imagine their white blood cells breeding as rabbits. All fine if you have the gift of imagination and concentration required to hold such creativity in your mind.

I DON'T.

I recognised that from day one. I do not have a powerfully imaginative mind but I do believe my body is a powerful and effective machine. No doubt about that, so when I attain the meditative state I describe in Chapter 5, I visualise my body as a gleaming engine. It is not inventive. Indeed the western mechanistic approach to medicine, 'body part broken let's go in and fix it' encourages me to think in a mechanistic way when I consider the being that I am.

I am the machine of me. My arteries and veins, and nerves, are wires of varying thickness, sheathed in toughened plastic rather than myelin. My muscles and sinews and ligaments, I see as a net of thick cord and rope. My bones and joints, are a series of drive shafts and props. My organs, steel boxes with inspection chambers I can open, to look inside, just like opening up a gear box. My brain is the electronic circuit board of any modern car. (Come on, you didn't think I would visualise myself as a 1920's model T Ford!).

The inspiration for my mechanistic imagery was a torso that sits on a plinth in my dining room; this quite brilliant model of a woman depicted as machine helps me travel within. It is for this reason it appears on the cover of this book (17).

Side by side with this artistic image I studied an anatomical chart.

Have you ever done that? Many brilliant textbooks on anatomy are readily available but if you want clarity and exceptional graphic representation I would suggest that you buy the best oversize book on human anatomy in colour you can afford.

I tell you, consideration of an anatomical textbook alone will make you think differently about the manner in which you exist. The food you put in to your mouth. The toxins you include as a matter of course in your habitual life routine. I bet as a reflex action the amount you spend on a bottle of wine increases. Why fill your gut with chemical ridden substances that will damage the stomach lining and stun the cells of your brain when you can drink organic wine or wine laden with fruit that has not been sprayed in chemicals or made to ferment at speed as a result of acids thrown in to the vat?

I assure you connecting with your physical self every day will be the beginning of a new way of living.

So let us begin.

Let us look now at how to apply the tools I believe in: how to make each separate feted technique work in unity as one combined therapy that will if you believe in it alter the way you experience the rest of your life.

CHAPTER FIVE

THE RITUAL

THE PROCESS

This chapter can be your reference guide if you wish it to be, but remember the Ritual I perform is not a set of commands, I am not a drill major, it is simpler to show how my Ritual is carried out by including photographs of my performance than to include lengthy explanation, and it is simpler to explain, than to say;

'I perform this daily Ritual but I cannot really describe it'.

In consequence, I attempt to describe it here but feel free to use this chapter only for insight or as a guide to creating your own framework to give shape to a Ritual personal to yourself.

The essential aim of my Ritual is to take control of my health and the shape my body is in, by taking control of the information my brain processes and the messages and information communicated as a result of such processing to my body. It is effectively a rewiring of thought to eradicate any existing negative wiring of thoughts and beliefs that may be responsible for emotional or physical set back or decline.

It is necessary when performing the Ritual to bathe the whole of the body, every organ, muscle, nerve ending, and bone in positivity. The structures of the body should literally be steeped in positive thought.

I don't confine this attitude of showering myself in positivity to the 45 or so minutes of my day in which I perform my Ritual. I find as my Ritual has developed I am more and more aware of the life giving nature of positive energy. I now stop, if for only a minute, at random points of my day, to take a 'positive shower'. It is so easy and it is always beneficial. If I am walking, or sitting in my home, or standing in the garden I turn my thoughts inwards, clench up every muscle in my body and my face and feel positive energy drawn from outside my being to within me. I hold the positive emotion, feel it flow through me and then release every muscle and say to myself,

' I am awesome. I feel awesome and I am awesome'.

It is not egotism. It is an act of thanks. It is a way of reminding myself of the marvel of the human form and the body that I have and the potential I contain.

What is the point of the converse, of wallowing in self – misery and self –criticism?

There is no point. It is pointless. Within weeks of performing the Ritual, if nothing else has occurred, one thing will have changed. You will have become your own biggest fan! And believe me that alone is good for your health.

There is no point at all in negative thought. One negative thought leads to another, which leads to a change in emotional state, which leads to a change in attitude, which leads to two things, negative action or worse, in action. Negative patterns of thinking are destructive, they lead to action which is destructive of the self or of others or even worse, in action, doing nothing with the negativity generated other than harbouring it and storing it within, which in my opinion is one sure route to allowing in disease and decline.

So as a precursor to performance of the Ritual consider your thoughts and if they are negative, eliminate them, every one of them. Take each negative thought in turn and address it, release it, don't even attempt to connect with it.

When I perform my Ritual I am trying to saturate the whole of my body with this positivity I describe by connecting mentally with the organs and structures within me and thanking each for the job that is being done. I want my liver, kidneys, heart and every structure I have to feel appreciated, to be congratulated for performing optimally.

I am ready for my average reader to believe at this point I 'have lost my marbles', or, 'I am existing in cloud cuckoo land', but in my opinion, 'cloud cuckoo land' is not such a bad place to live.

Take a look at the back cover of this book. That is me kite surfing at the age of 70. I would not have had this photograph at age 65. I would not as a younger man have been ready for the physical and mental challenge of manipulating a kite, with a twelve foot span, on the waves of the sea, while balancing on what can be considered as an over sized skate board. I would not have been ready because all I was ready for was ageing and a narrowed, less active, lifestyle.

I absolutely believe, through communication with my inner self, by journeying within and beginning a conversation with the body that I have, I have not only, for the first time in my life, realised the complexity and potential I possess under my skin. I have through my mantra of appreciation and expression of gratitude for the job the structures within me are doing, restored vitality energy and youthfulness.

I totally believe it is possible to create a mental connection between the brain and every part of the body and to hold a conversation between mind and every body part. I believe and so it happens and it works.

What are we talking about? Is it the confounding elephant in the room, the 'placebo effect'? I think that it is. It is either that or it is something much more advanced which neither I, nor any scientist involved in the study of mankind, is as yet able to explain. Let's remind ourselves of the many theories

I skirt over in Chapter 3 and remind ourselves also that the mystery of what is really within us and what it is within our potential to achieve is not fully resolved.

I do not propose to solve it by setting out the basis of my Ritual, if anything, the effectiveness of my Ritual complicates even further the conundrum, of why, on occasion, the body acts as it does to reverse decline, repel disease and repair itself, as a reaction, it would seem, to a belief held in the potential for recovery to occur. A belief that can only be formed by information the brain is given to deal with.

Think about that; choose your thoughts carefully, as I choose mine. I brainwash myself into believing that my Ritual can do all that I say that it can and a circular response ensues. My brain reacts to the good news every organ, bone, blood vessel, nerve ending is in optimal condition and my body flourishes. I see the results obtained from my therapeutic programme, which in turn endorses my belief in its effectiveness, validating for my brain the result I predict.

Before I set out for you what my Ritual involves, a word of warning, the explanation given of my Ritual process includes the terms 'meditative state' and 'mindfulness'.

If some years ago I had picked up a book that told me the key to better health, longevity, raised energy, youthfulness and prolonged vitality required me to create a 'meditative state' I would have immediately set it down. I was not a meditator. Meditation was something Buddhists did in far off countries where the weather was better and every one had time on their hands. Meditation was not for me. So let me tell you two things. Firstly performance of the Ritual requires the performer to attain a meditative state and secondly and most importantly any one practising my Ritual will find their way to this state naturally without any effort, until to meditate becomes as natural as switching the kettle on to make a cup of tea.

You do not have to dedicate months or years of your life to learning the art of meditation. I have gone before you and I have tried meditation as one of a regime of therapies I grasped at in the hope of becoming a 'better', more fulfilled, less irascible human being. It didn't work. I stayed wide- eyed in class listening to the traffic noise or the central heating. I could not take myself within. If I had spent the last ten years attempting to meditate I would never have managed to alter the nature of the conversation I have each day with my inner being. I would remain a total failure as a meditator and I would no doubt think bringing myself in to a state of mindfulness was beyond my grasp.

Now by a totally unintended route, I 'meditate', for almost an hour a day. I perform my Ritual 'mindfully', as this is the only way it can be performed, if it is to be effective. So let me change the vocabulary and see if I can carry you with me. When I describe entering a meditative state, I am describing the act of lying down upon my bed, stilling my mind and concentrating upon what I am doing.

I focus on the task in hand. I connect with the shape of myself on the inside. That is not complicated. Try it. Lay your hand upon your chest and locate your beating heart. Think of the shape of the organ your heart is, beating a short distance from your fingertips. With the help of the anatomy text –book, I suggested you purchase, lay your hands on other parts of your body. Locate your kidney and your liver, your lungs your spleen. Run your hands along the length of the major bones in your thigh. It is not hard is it? Just concentrate. Concentrate upon how you look on the inside and recognise the extraordinary nature of your physical being. Be impressed, over awed, inspired and be grateful.

That is it. That is the first step towards creation of your own daily Ritual, recognising the amazing nature of your physical self and the power, gifts and ability, you as a human being possess.

WHAT THE RITUAL INVOLVES

1. The placing of the fingers on the body to correspond with the positioning of the organ or structure within the body to be worked upon. The application of therapeutic touch to target and guide thoughts and affirmations that are held in the mind to the task of rejuvenation, maintenance or repair of the body part targeted.
2. Total mindfulness, that is to say, concentration upon and engagement with the task in hand, which is to praise and congratulate the body part, structure or system worked upon for the job that is being done.
3. Visualisation of the body part, structure, bodily system or organ, in good health, fully functioning and effective and as new and polished and clear of disease, as the images in my text book of anatomy.
4. I see my body as an engine. Each body part or structure is visualised as a powerful and dynamic part of a glistening well maintained whole. Each part works integrally as part of a shining and polished machine. The material of the machine I imagine is indestructible, able to run and interact with every other part within the engine of myself for at least a thousand years. I would stress any imagery that persuades an individual mind to believe in the power of a body to direct itself towards health and longevity will be effective.
5. The most powerful part of my Ritual is the on going dialogue, my conversation with my organs and every other body part, creates between my body and my mind. I repeatedly, but silently affirm, what fantastic shape my body is in, how marvellous a machine my body is.

This system of silent communication, built from a series of affirmations repeated on a daily basis, can I believe, persuade my body of only one thing: it is magnificent.

I did not set out to create a programme, which involved targeted meditation, therapeutic touch, visualisation and affirmation. I set out to begin a conversation with my self. To communicate to my inner being the gratitude I held in my mind for the job that my body was doing. All evolved from that point and it was from the point of my Ritual's success that I began to try to understand more about mindful meditation, visualisation, touch therapy and affirmation. I came at the theory from an effort to understand the practice rather than the other way around. I want to let everyone know this, so that all those who have never before considered themselves drawn to activities such as meditation, affirmation, positive thinking, visualisation, do not set this book aside but give the Ritual a chance.

I began a conversation with my inner being which I could only achieve by switching my perspective from the world around me and focusing my thoughts within, on my insides, on my cells and tissues, on the man that I was beneath my skin.

That was the beginning, but you will realise from incorporation in to this book of the 'Everyday Face Lift' and 'The Recumbent Gym', that I soon saw the Ritual could not only benefit my inner being but also my external self. The same technique was involved, just a different conversation, a different belief, directed to improve skin tone, facial appearance and musculature.

I am now convinced after years of Ritual performance that my Ritual has further to evolve. I am a beginner and we are at the beginning of knowledge. I am still learning how best to develop and benefit from my intervention in the continual conversation, taking place between my body and my mind.

I believe through the practice of my Ritual I interfere with this conversation. I say more about this in Chapter 10 when dealing with the work of Candace Pert. By altering the thoughts I hold and shaping my beliefs I provide new facts for my brain to process. This, 'rewiring' changes the outcome a normal, uninterrupted, undirected, conversation between my body and my mind can achieve.

The uninterrupted dialogue created by my mind, would I believe, not be as positive, as focused, or as optimistic, as the newly created dialogue, the Ritual directs. The normal information exchange between my body and my mind, generated not only by bio-chemical activity, but by my un marshalled thoughts, sentiments and emotional reactions to events within my life, would be less positive, less able to persuade my ever receptive consciousness, that I was in good health, invincible, capable of rejuvenation, capable indeed of living, for an indefinite period, an unlimited life.

The Ritual to me now is almost second nature. I could not think of living out the rest of my life with out taking myself within my consciousness to join in the conversation on going between my body and my mind. I now every day, am driven to say my piece, emphasise the truth, as I see it, of the potential I have, the health I can possess, of the stimulation and excitement awaiting me in my many future years.

Trust me, you have to try it. Within a period of months, if not weeks, you will not believe the ease with which a person can connect with their on going mind-body dialogue to completely re write the script of their own life.

3. METHOD

My Ritual is intended to energise and restore my body and mind. Each exercise requires the following staged procedure for full benefit to be gained.

STAGE ONE

Take yourself within. I know only one method and that is to close my eyes and listen to the world around me.

It may be silent or it may be full of intrusion from activity outside my home, caused by others living their lives or caused by others within my home living their lives. Sounds are of interest not an irritation when the Ritual is performed and the Ritual can be performed despite noise external to your mind. The right state of mind for performance of the Ritual comes through concentration. The act of shutting the eyes is an act of separation from your outside life. With your eyes closed you can concentrate in a different way.

Some minutes of simply lying flat or sitting still with your eyes closed should cause you to experience a sense of detachment from your external world. You will be aware of the world you are part of but you should be aware of something else, your inner state. Your body should feel like a space inhabited, a mechanism for living you are perhaps for the first time viewing from this altered perspective.

In this state of mind I make contact with my body on the inside. I imagine my body as a highly polished powerful and effective machine. I have said choice of imagery is a personal matter. You may prefer not to visualise but simply connect in the manner I have described earlier by simply focusing upon the body that you have and the shape of the structures within it. Making the connection is not hard it just takes an act of concentration.

As you concentrate consider the magnificence and complexity of the body you possess. Form a thought and recognise the thought forming. It can be anything.

How fast your heart is beating.

How deep your breathing is.

Recognise yourself thinking about the body that you have and recognise the separation of thought and your physical body your thought concerns. Recognise when you close your eyes you are in control of the thoughts that you form and hold. Sit and allow your brain to send a message to your toe. Large toe left foot. Tell the toe to move.

Experience the creation and delivery of the message. Do not open your eyes.

Realise what just happened. You formed a thought, a message was sent from brain to body and your toe, as directed moved. Realise the power within yourself and realise the gift of this inner consciousness to direct and alter the physical form you possess.

You can alter your perspective to bring your focus from your exterior life, to your life lived on the inside of your body. It will not be usual for you to do this but it is possible any time you wish to concentrate upon the relationship between your mind and body and the manner in which they work together. In this state of inward concentration you can experience the body in a different way. As often as you wish you can direct your mind to focus on a particular body part.

With only a little practice you will find you can enter a different mental plane, a plane of detachment by simply stilling your mind and closing your eyes.

After only minutes of sitting contemplatively in this way, separating physicality from consciousness, you should be aware that you are seeing yourself from another perspective. This may be the first time in your life you have ever considered yourself in this way. Try to arrive at this level of awareness of your conscious and physical self every day.

When you have attained this necessary perspective, focus on the extraordinary power of your mind to direct the body that you have. Consider the extent of your physical body, neutrally and objectively. Do not open your eyes. Consider yourself from within. Create an image of yourself in your mind sitting in the chair you are sitting in or lying upon your bed and view yourself in the mental image you create as you may regard a stranger on a bus.

WHY?

Because as long as this sense of detachment from your physical body is maintained you are in a deeply meditative state which allows you to communicate with your sub-conscious brain. The images you present to your sub-conscious in this state will be lived out in your conscious world of physical existence in the days and years to follow.

What we carry in our sub- conscious we manifest. Don't ask me why, I am a beginner at this. Perhaps it is because we hold in our sub-conscious brain all the powerful thoughts, beliefs, desires and weaknesses of our life. Perhaps it is only by communication with our sub-conscious we can go in and sort out the things that without our knowledge are affecting the being that we are, our day to day health, the way in which we live.

The meditative state has an unknown power within it and it is within our individual gift to shift our mind to this meditative plane. We are all able to alter our perspective, to turn inwards upon our being, to direct the brain to change the emotions stored within us, emotions that unknown to us may be nurturing disease.

Thought impacts upon our cells; scientists have demonstrated this to be the case. Imagine therefore the power within the mind to straighten out our limiting beliefs of inevitable decay and to fill us instead with joyfulness and optimism about the future that is ours. Visualise yourself healthy, vigorous, and in synch with the energy of the universe and your attitude to illness will change. Visualise yourself empowered, energised and able to do anything, and I promise you, you will be.

I have no idea why this works.

If I could I would chat to the Dalai Lama and ask for some insights but I can't and so I will simply continue with my routine and try as I develop in experience to unravel what I am doing. One thing I am certain of, I would not trade my 45 minute daily Ritual for all the innovative anti-ageing pharmaceuticals presently in design. My Ritual for me is a better means of rejuvenating my being than any elixir that could exist.

Meditating is just another way of thinking. It is something we are never taught, but we could be. It is not something riddled with secrets or magic, it is easy and accessible and it allows access to a dimension of our self we rarely experience. This dimension that we rarely feel or appreciative is a place of power we still do not fully understand. I believe it makes all the limits upon human potential, proposed by scientists, medics and others, meaningless.

STAGE TWO

Do not panic.

The worst response you could have to endeavouring to act as I describe in Stage One is dejection because things did not work out.

Read the rest of this Chapter and then take a deep breath.

My Ritual is meant to be enjoyable. Out of it will develop your own Ritual for your life and it will become addictive, something you wish to engage in because of the break from stress it provides and the serenity it induces.

If having tried to meditate as I describe in Stage One you could not do it or are not there yet.

DO NOT BECOME IRRITATED OR FRUSTRATED
CERTAINLY DO NOT BECOME DOWNHEARTED

The state of mind the Ritual requires every human being on earth can create. It is not complicated it is simple. It is so simple that it is easy to try too hard, failing to realise, how accessible our ability to alter the manner in which we see ourselves is.

For those of you who are struggling, let us consider things again.

What happens when you close your eyes.

What did you see?

Nothing save a darkened space? Whiteness, greyness, nothingness, colour? Whatever is seen behind the eyes, counts. Hold the sensation of blankness, of separation from your exterior life and relax, this is your fourth dimension, the dimension within yourself.

It is upon this that I impose the image of the body as machine. I see my body and brain as a series of cogs and wheels and pivots and bars and chambers and boxes and grids and I relax into this imagery knowing that I am engineered to the highest specification and I am capable of anything. Holding this mechanised imagery in my mind I begin a series of silent affirmations, forming within my consciousness the thought my mind needs to hear. I do not verbalise the affirmations that I make, if anything I feel them. I know this act of silent affirmation is powerful. On occasion I can feel my body respond as the statements are formed in my consciousness and processed by my mind.

I AM AWESOME

I AM IN GREAT SHAPE

I WORK AS WELL TODAY AS I DID WHEN I WAS 28

I WILL REMAIN FIT AND VIGOROUS AND ABLE THROUGHOUT EVERY DECADE THAT REMAINS OF MY LIFE

ANYTHING I CHOOSE TO DO I HAVE THE ABILITY TO DO

I AM THE MOST AMAZING OUTSTANDING PIECE OF ENGINEERING AND I HAVE THE POWER TO MAINTAIN MYSELF OR RESTORE MYSELF TO THIS AMAZING STATE

I believe affirmations are powerful even when not verbalised. All that matters is at the point the affirmation is formed it is believed. As I have stated a number of times, once a fact is believed it has power, sufficient to work upon our psyche, to change our responses, the way in which we act and the shape we are in.

Affirming when meditating, I am persuaded, does the same thing, as Monsieur Coue's pronouncements to his patients, but more directly, more powerfully, as all of our mental processes are unfolding in our 'closed in state', the state we create when we concentrate and shift our perspective inwards.

Affirm the facts you wish to make manifest, silently, over and over again, a least a dozen times. Know the truth of the facts you are placing in to your consciousness, and,

THAT'S IT, that is the end of the second stage of my Ritual and the end of preparing the body and the brain to be receptive to the work you are now going to do.

DO NOT OPEN YOUR EYES

Stay relaxed and position your fingertips upon the first section of your body you wish to work upon.

STAGE THREE

THERAPIES COMBINED

Each exercise I take you through should be performed with the brain in the state of concentration described and the mind focused upon the part of the body a particular exercise concerns. Either place the finger tips directly on the area to be worked upon or in the case of exercises dealing with deep structures or organs within the body, place the finger tips on an area of skin proximate to the location of the relevant organ, structure or system the exercise concerns.

I am sure within weeks you will come to understand much more about your anatomy. In the brief learning period use the purchased anatomy text -book for reference. As you work upon a particular area of the body create your own mental image of this body part as it would appear in the best of health.

As I take you through my Ritual exercises I suggest some images for various body parts but I encourage you to use your own created imagery if you can. I believe there is even greater prospect of therapeutic mind body communication if each individual visualises a body part in terms of their own psyche and the emotions contained within it.

Stimulate each body part using therapeutic touch as I describe and create an affirmation that says something about the body part, system or organ worked upon that gives thanks for the job that the part or structure does. Express the firm belief that in future the job the body part, system or structure does will be done brilliantly, without any obstruction or problem getting in the way.

TO BEGIN

I begin with the lymph system. You may wish to start elsewhere. In Chapter 7 I include a number of exercises for various areas of the body. You may not wish to perform a full Ritual, you may wish to pick and choose and so feel free to skip ahead to an exercise shown for a part of the body that is troubling you at present or for an area you consider important. If you are following my Ritual the initial part of your own Ritual will be dedicated to working upon the lymph system to stimulate the flow of lymph around the body.

Our lymph system is a major part of our immune system.

When did you last pay attention to your own lymph system?

Never? Is the response I imagine I would receive from the majority of my readers. Or from those even more disconnected from the body they possess, an enquiry,

'My lymph system, what's that, and where is it ?'

Let's take a look at that.

If you are to derive maximum benefit from a daily performance of the Ritual it is useful to understand where groups of lymph nodes are situated around the body, to know the job that they do and how the Ritual endeavours to apply itself to the maintenance and efficient working of the entire lymph system. If you have anatomical diagrams of the body available to you, now may be a good time to have a look at an illustration or photograph of the connected circuit of lymph nodes in the human body in an effort to understand just what it is that the lymph system does.

Once you are comfortable with the concept of the movement of lymph and have an idea in your mind as to where the groups of lymph nodes within the body are situated we can move on to Chapter 6.

CHAPTER SIX

THE RITUAL FOR THE LYMPH SYSTEM

I begin my Ritual with a set of exercises which are targeted upon the lymph nodes. I believe the lymphatic system to be one of the systems within the body most likely to benefit from stimulation through therapeutic touch, and one of the most powerful systems we rely upon to maintain our body in good shape and to restore good health in the event our health is in decline.

WHAT IS THE LYMPH SYSTEM?

The lymph system is an elaborate system of 600 – 700 lymph nodes dispersed around the body. I enclose a diagram of the lymph system at Fig 6.1.

I believe we do not pay sufficient attention to our lymph system. The reason it seems is that most of us do not know what the lymph system does, or how it works or the important role it plays in sustaining good health.

When the importance of good lymphatic flow to sustained immunity and protection from disease, was explained to me, I had no doubt at all when creating my Ritual I should include a set of exercises to focus upon the areas of my body in which lymph nodes are concentrated, (the arm pits, neck and groin,).

The purpose of this chapter is to demonstrate the Ritual exercises I apply to my lymph system. If you wish to skip this chapter and move ahead to the principal Ritual exercises go ahead, but before you make your decision I should mention one important thing. Since the time I have incorporated the exercises within this chapter in to my Ritual I have not succumbed to a cold or virus or suffered an infection of any kind. It may be just a coincidence or it may be a consequence of the attention I have paid to a previously under appreciated system within my body.

I leave the choice with you, choose to learn and practice the group of exercises intended to stimulate the lymph system, or take your chances of succumbing to each and every virus that circulates in our society and move on.

METHOD

Follow the preparatory steps for performance of the Ritual I set out in Chapter 5, when describing what my Ritual involves.

I find it helpful when working on my lymph system to hold an image of a rubber ball hand pump in my mind. The type of pump used to inflate an air mattress. When the ball is squeezed it expels air and when pressure upon it is relaxed a suction motion allows it to fill with air. I hold this image of a rubber air pump in my mind as I image the lymph nodes under my fingers filling with and releasing lymph fluid.

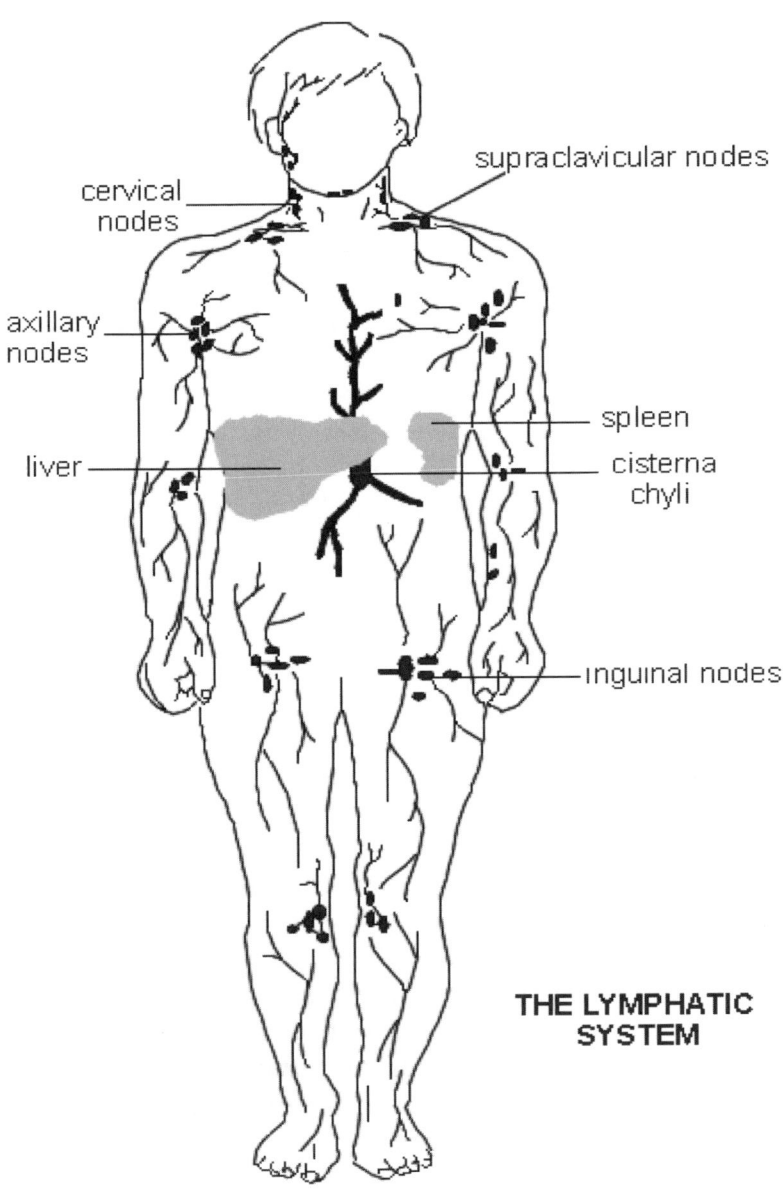

cervical nodes

supraclavicular nodes

axillary nodes

liver

spleen

cisterna chyli

inguinal nodes

THE LYMPHATIC SYSTEM

Fig 6.1

THE NECK (1)

In order to stimulate the lymph system I begin work on my neck as a large concentration of lymph nodes and glands are situated in this area.

I place my fingertips in the position shown in photograph Fig 6.2

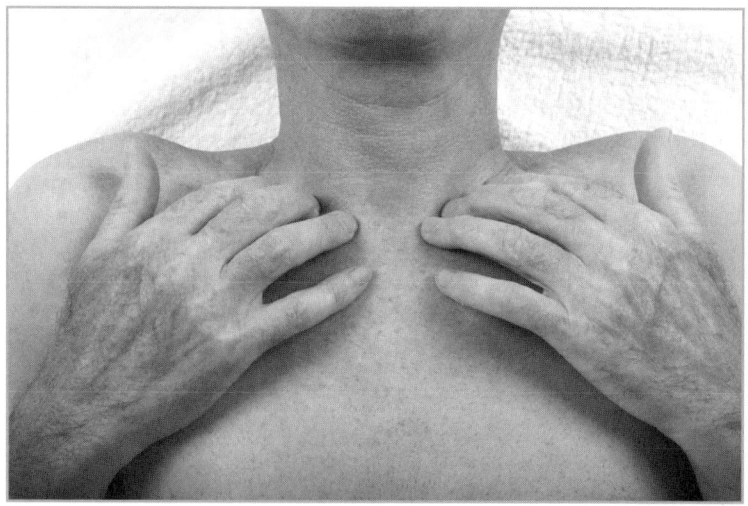

Fig 6.2

When I am in a state of mindfulness, that is of quiet concentration upon my inner self I apply therapeutic touch, with my finger -tips in the position demonstrated.

I place the finger tips of each hand on the edge of the collar- bone, either side of the clavicle, letting the finger tips slide in to the soft tissues slightly behind the collar bone. With the finger- tips in this position I tense the lower muscles in my neck. You will feel your finger- tips lift. Release the neck muscle and the finger-tips will gently sink behind the collar bone. Be gentle with your movements, be mindful and hold each movement for one second.

Use the image I have provided of the lymph gland in this area working as a pump. Imagine the pump working as your fingertips palpate your skin and imagine lymph flowing into a pipe attached to the visualised pump. See the lymph flowing downwards along the tubes leading from the pump. This strongly held visual image should coincide with your action of directing lymphatic fluid with your fingertips, from your neck, downwards in to the venus angle where it returns to the circulatory system.

Silently affirm to your sub-conscious that your lymph system is in good shape and doing a great job and that all the toxins of the body are eradicated from every cell as a result of the good work the lymph system is doing. Congratulate your lymph system for working so well.

NECK (2)

We then move on to the neck and to the area around the ears. With the hands and fingers as shown in fig 6.3. Slowly stroke down with the fingers towards the clavicle area, imagining gently moving the lymph just below the surface of the skin.

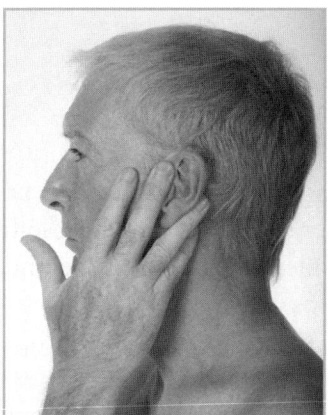

Fig 6.3

THE JAW BONE

I then move to stimulate the lymph nodes just under the jaw-bone as shown in Fig 6.4. Using the right hand I gently move the second and third fingers of my left hand beneath the lower edge of the jaw bone, moving from the chin to below the ear.

I visualise the flow of lymph towards the outer neck and then down towards the clavicle.

Repeat this movement 20 times on each side of the jaw.

Remember to concentrate upon the task you are engaged with. Be mindful. Be grateful. During every moment celebrate the work of your lymph system.

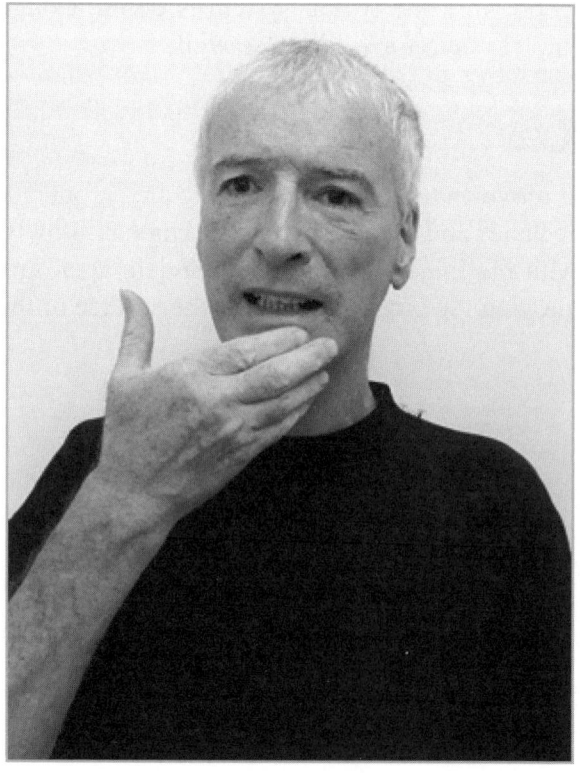

Fig 6.4

THE GROIN AND THE LEGS

Next we stimulate the lymph nodes in the groin or inguinal area. Place the fingers of the right hand across the crease of the right groin as demonstrated in 6.5. This should place your right hand approximately in position with your lymph nodes. Flex the muscles in this area so that you can feel the movement through your fingertips and visualise the nodes beneath your fingers. With each flex and relax of the muscles visualise the lymph nodes as a pump. Visualise the pump working to pump lymphatic fluid, with great effect, to the lymph nodes in the area of the torso and abdomen. Affirm the benefits of the work the lymph system is doing, repeat 20 times on each side of the groin.

To finish this exercise I move the lymph from the ankle down the leg to the groin. To achieve this I raise the right leg. I gently stroke the surface tissue of the leg from the ankle to the groin using my fingertips. I visualise lymph fluid moving down the leg and affirm what a great job my lymph system is doing. I repeat the action on the left leg.

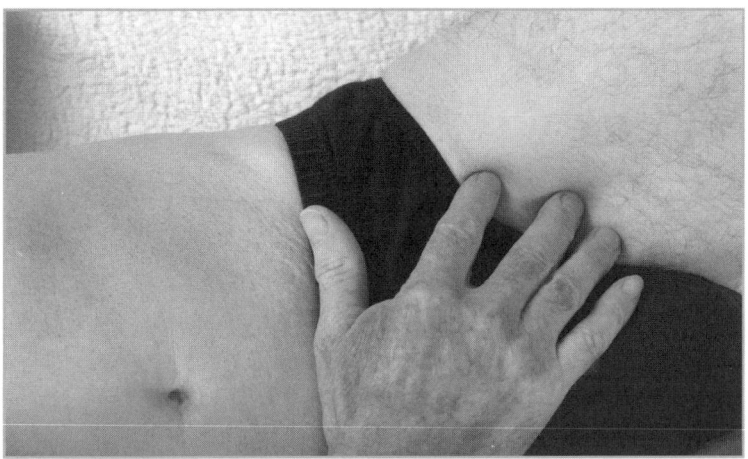

Fig 6.5

STERNUM

The next area I work to stimulate is just below the sternum, beneath the bottom of the rib cage. This is an area with considerable lymphatic presence and it is also the location of the gall bladder. Place the fingertips as shown in photograph 6.6.

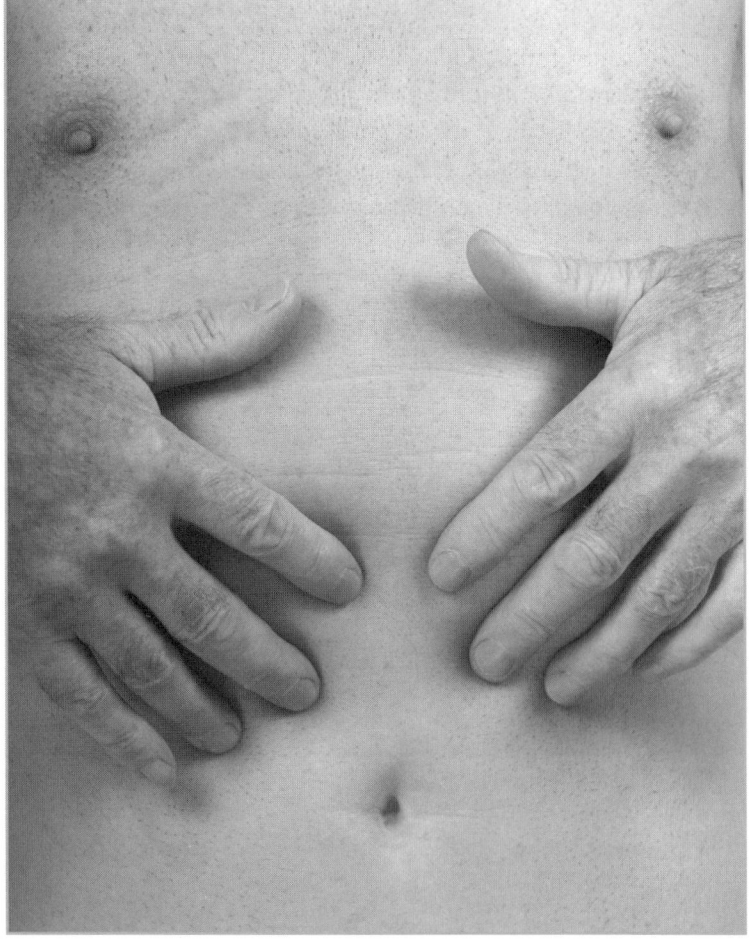

Fig 6.6

Perform the exercise in exactly the same way. Your mind will now be in a state of concentration or mindfulness. Your sub-conscious will be filled with an awareness of your inner body. In this mindful state you should have a keen awareness of your physical body and the connection between this body and the mind. This mind –body link and separation should be felt more acutely than in your day- to - day life. Visualise a group of pumps working in unison as there are many lymph nodes in this area. See each pump working and see liquid flowing in to pipework connected to the pumps. Affirm to yourself that the whole process is working well. Be grateful for the state your lymph system is in. Allow a feeling of gratitude and love to flow between your mind and the lymph nodes located in the area of the sternum. Affirm your belief that for decades to come the good work done by the lymph system will continue.

THE ARM PITS

I address the lymph system in the arm - pit area as shown in fig 6.7. I place the fingers of my right hand flat on the tissues of the left arm - pit. I tuck my fingers in to my arm-pit and feel them against the chest wall. I gently squeeze my left arm against the fingers of my right hand. I breathe in and feel the muscular movement as muscles contract beneath my fingers. On each flex of my fingers, I imagine the lymph nodes in this area working. I visualise the lymph node taking up lymph fluid and filling. I then relax the muscles I am working with and imagine lymph fluid being released from the node and pumped up towards the neck. I repeat the contraction of my muscles 20 times. I then repeat the exercise by placing my left hand in the same position under my right arm with the fingers of my left hand pressed in to my right arm - pit.

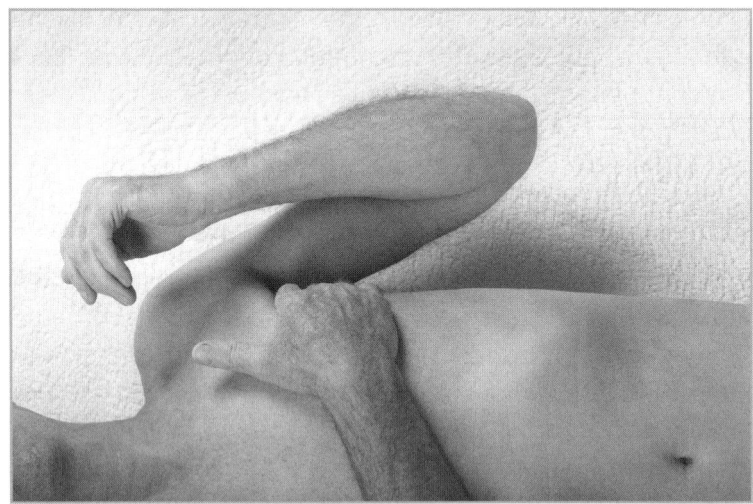

Fig 6.7

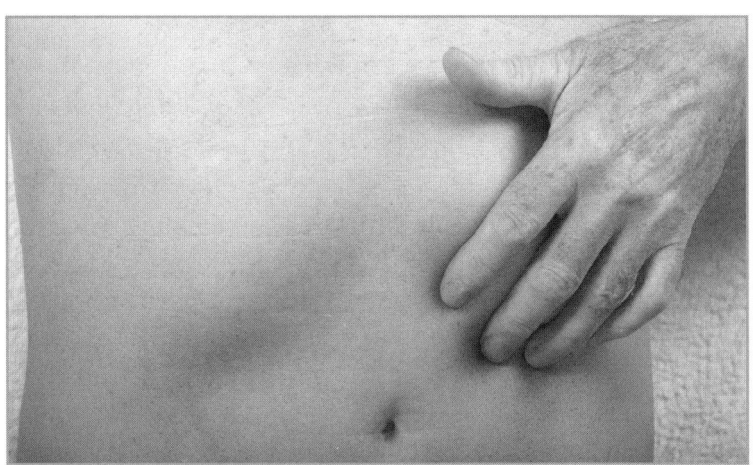

Fig 6.8

THE SPLEEN

The spleen is one of the principal organs involved in lymphatic drainage. Our aim with this exercise is to stimulate the spleen and optimise splenic function.

Apply pressure to the tissues proximate to the spleen by placing the fingertips of the left hand under the central lower ledge of the left rib cage as shown in fig 6.8.

The spleen acts as a filter for old red blood cells and as a gland organ in which blood can be stored to be used by the body in an emergency. The spleen is not necessary to sustain life but it plays a part in sustaining good immunity, creating antibodies and repelling certain bacteria such as those responsible for meningitis. If the spleen is damaged or failing to perform, the body's immunity to disease is weakened.

You will understand, by this point, that applying therapeutic touch as in Fig 6.8 and squeezing the muscles in the tissue surrounding the spleen engages the attention of the brain upon the task of awakening and regenerating the spleen and congratulating it upon the job that it is doing.

At all times direct the emotion of love and gratitude from the brain to the spleen.

Apply therapeutic touch. Pump the tissues up and down at least 20 times.

Relax.

That is it. The group of exercises I have taken you through are enough to maintain and energise the lymph system. Commit to working on the lymph system in this way and within days you should feel a benefit. I felt less tired, more energised, and was undoubtedly more active.

It is hard now to separate the consequences of the lymph system exercises from the general health benefits the Ritual delivers but I absolutely believe without the exercises targeted upon lymph nodes my Ritual would be substantially less effective. We have considered the massive power in belief and my belief in the effectiveness of the lymph node exercises is in many respects self fulfilling.

Time to move on to the rest of the body and to the Ritual exercises for the main organs, the brain, skeletal and nervous systems, set out in Chapter 7.

CHAPTER SEVEN

THE RITUAL EXERCISES

Next time you are in the shower take a good look at the body you have. Run your hand over your shin, along your thigh. Feel your skin and think about the job that it does. One coating of skin for your entire lifetime, that unknown to you is replacing itself every two to four weeks, toughening, wrinkling, staying smooth, depending on the job you do and how you care for the substance that it is. One impermeable layer to keep you dry, warm, contained. A huge jacket under which your blood runs and your bones are held in place. Do you ever think about yourself in this way? Do you ever connect with the absolutely amazing entity that your body is?

In creating my Ritual I have endeavoured to create a programme that will impact upon the circuitry of the most ingenious work of engineering ever achieved. If you realise only one thing from reading this chapter realise this, any therapeutic ritual presented with the challenge my Ritual faces is not going to deliver results over night. In fact without a massive shift in our mindset and a willingness to break through the shell of ourselves, to the unknown place within, it is not going to deliver at all.

We have all we need within us to heal restore and regenerate the body we possess. We can re-gain the vitality of our past, regenerate our cells and live for a very long time, but we can only do this by bringing our focus to rest in a dimension in which we normally do not exist. I think it profoundly ironic that by an act of concentration upon our inner self we change fundamentally the capability that we have to connect with a greater energy beyond ourselves, an energy that has the power within it to rejuvenate and enrich.

I consider when the mind accepts an outcome with unquestioning belief, believing in the outcome sought, profoundly, unshakeably and absolutely, to the extent that only one outcome is possible, something happens within us, something extraordinary and inexplicable which creates an environment for self healing.

The important thing is to connect with the being that you are in a way you are simply unused to doing. It is time to make your mind focus upon the visceral, the messy, the blood and guts and structures of yourself.

Some people make the right connection, not in the way of my Ritual, not by imposing a therapeutic regime upon their life, but living their entire life therapeutically. Those who live to be 103 still walking up hills, enjoying the view, out pacing younger men (1), have most certainly engaged their mind in maintaining their body, unwittingly unleashing from within them what it takes to maintain vitality energy and seemingly perpetual youth.

The Ritual is my way of accessing the gift I have, that everyone has, of managing and orchestrating health and self repair. I do not suggest it is the only way or a complete answer to the conundrum of enduring wellness, but for those who have not a clue about how to tackle the onslaught of ageing it is a pretty good start.

I include in this chapter the Ritual exercises I perform on all of the major organs of my body. I perform these exercises after I complete my daily work on my lymph system. The lymph system exercises when perfected take no more than ten minutes to complete. I target the principal organs of my body in the performance of my Ritual.

It would have been possible to identify other body parts and to work upon them but I do not have the time. I conclude this chapter with an exercise for the brain. I call this exercise 'the pituitary shower'. This is an exercise intended to benefit the whole body. My Ritual has to work to support a life. It cannot be so long and drawn out and complicated that the average man or woman simply has no time to perform it. I provide enough information in Chapters 5 to 9 to allow any one to understand how to create an individual exercise for a bodily structure, system or part this book does not cover. My Ritual as created picks and chooses the essential organs I wish to stimulate. I believe I am doing my body a great service and I believe my Ritual will reward me well. If you begin the Ritual in a position of ill health target your own exercises to the body part or system you consider needs them the most.

Be patient. Do not seek immediate results. Perform the exercises I describe repeatedly and with commitment and beneficial results will come.

For each exercise follow this sequence of actions:

1. Relax
2. Close your eyes and concentrate to the point where your perception of yourself alters from the person that you are on the outside to the person that you are within. Recognise your mind is in communication with your body. Experience this communication. Fix your mind upon different body parts, upon the nervous system, upon the skeleton. Appreciate the alteration of focus as your mind settles on differing body parts, moving with your thoughts and the images you hold in your imagination. Hold your concentration within, upon this new, no doubt unexplored dimension of yourself.

Remain with this altered perspective, enjoy existing within your fourth dimension.

3. Breathe deeply, rhythmically, peacefully.

4. Create in your brain the image you wish to use to portray yourself in a perfect state of health. Choose an image that shows you as vital and energised, effective and vigorous, an image that symbolises for you, your body in perfect condition. Move from this whole body image to part of the visualised image only, the part which represents the part of your body you wish the Ritual to work upon.

5. Place your fingertips upon the area of your body to be worked upon and let your mind be directed by therapeutic touch to focus upon this area. Apply therapeutic touch. Imagine the body part, system or structure, energised and restored. Silently affirm the great job the targeted part of the body is doing and the great shape it is in.

6. Try to hold praise, gratitude and thanks as your most prevalent emotion throughout each exercise. When you apply your fingertips to any body area feel compassion, love, tenderness and positivity flood from your mind to the body part, system, or structure you are working with.

1. ABDOMEN

Place the hands as shown in fig 7.1.

Pull in the stomach and flex the abdominal muscles under the fingertips. Hold in your mind an awareness of the tissues and structures between spine and surface of the skin right up from the centre of your being to the tips of your fingers. Connect with the motion of your fingers, feel the energy of the motion you create, with the therapeutic touch you apply, pass through the fingertips to the skin, to the deep tissues, muscle, and fibres beneath.

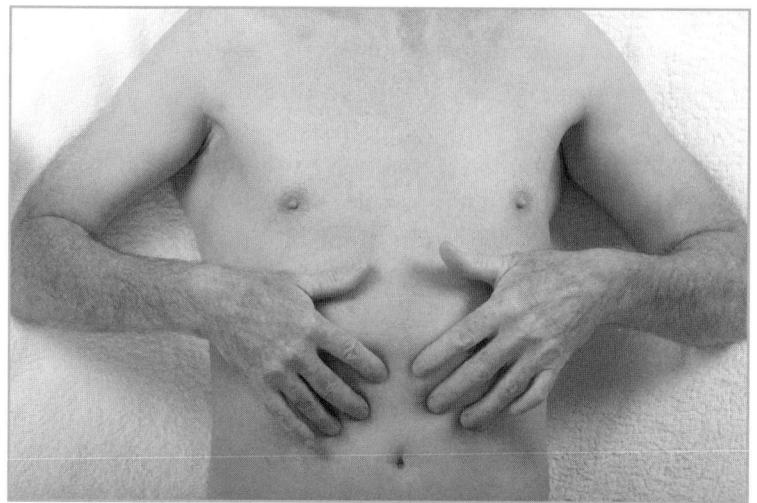

Fig 7.1

Feel your body respond to the therapeutic touch. Imagine the deepest muscles within you contracting and releasing. Feel the gratitude of your body as you visualise your body responding to the touch therapy. Be mindful of this response, be mindful of the connection between your fingertips and the very centre of your being.

Create an image that depicts for you your stomach working perfectly.

Start with your anatomy textbook if you have no idea what your stomach looks like.

Visualise a perfectly healthy stomach or impose an image from the full body metaphor you have created through imaging. My stomach is my petrol tank. It is full of fuel, which is being released and burned effectively to drive the engine of my body forward. The stomach walls are shiny and clean. The intestines are exhausts and pipework, shining chrome, shooting out flame as my digestive processes work and fuel the body that I have.

You may be working with entirely different imagery or you may be content to hold in your mind an image of a perfectly healthy stomach lifted directly from a coloured picture in your text book of anatomy.

Why not? If you have chosen a perfectly healthy stomach what better image could you impose in your brain?

Silently affirm that your stomach is in great shape and doing a great job and that everything it does, in taking in food, processing it and dispersing energy from nutrition to every other body part and system is recognised and appreciated. Connect with the job your stomach is doing and give full - hearted praise for the task.

Massage the skin as shown in fig7.1. Pump the tissues in the area shown with a slow pumping motion that holds the attention of your brain upon the task of energising the stomach. Press in and release finger tips from the area at least twenty times.

Move on.

2. THE RITUAL FOR THE KIDNEYS.

Immense benefit is to be gained by performing the Ritual on the outside of the body in the area of the kidneys. The kidneys are each about the size of a fist and are positioned near the centre of the back, just below the rib cage. The job of the kidneys is to filter the blood, to sift out water and waste, which leaves the body as urine. The kidneys are effectively a filtration plant. I imagine my kidneys doing an amazing job of filtering all toxins from my system. I affirm the amazing job that is being done. I flex the muscles in the area I am touching and I imagine powerful filtration plants working to expel all waste from my system.

I create this image while in a state of concentration or mindfulness. I apply therapeutic touch to the area of my back shown in fig 7.2. working one side of my body and then the next in the area of each kidney. I silently express my gratitude for the work each kidney is doing and I affirm that this work will continue to be done without any problem or need for intervention of any kind.

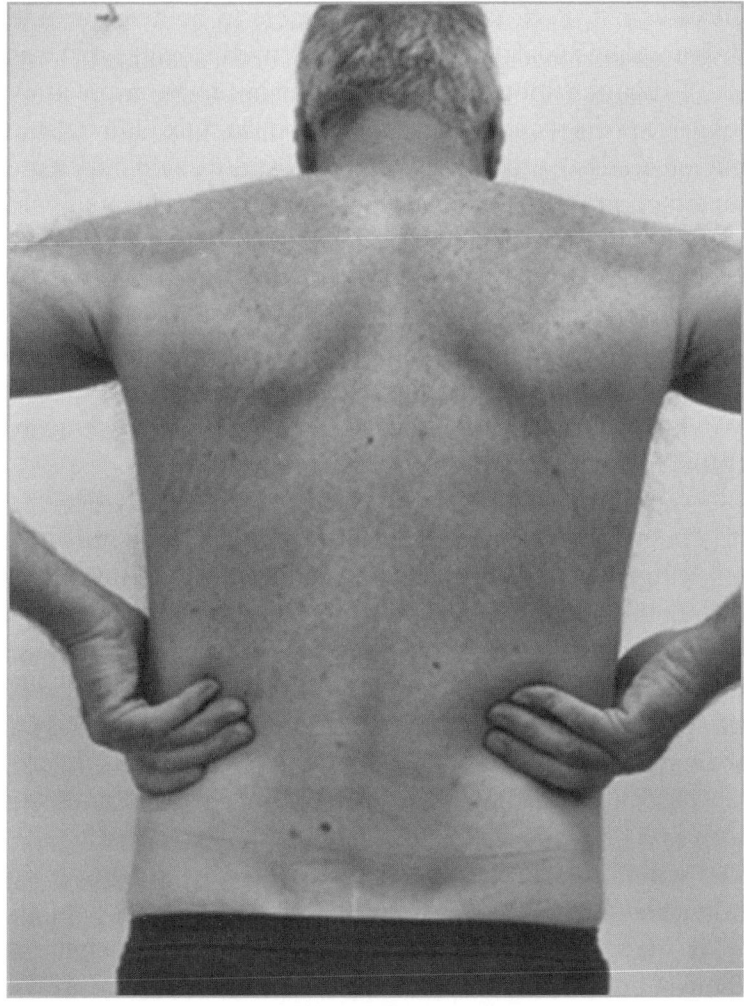

Fig 7.2

At present the Ritual I perform is thankfully preventive. I wish to maintain myself in good shape. I am not unwell. I do not suffer from any disease. You may say, well then, how can I tell you the Ritual delivers any benefit for my health when there is nothing wrong with me in the first place.

I would respond to this by stating the obvious. I am almost 70 years old. I am told I am vulnerable to both ageing and degeneration and decline. Indeed over twenty years ago I was told I required spinal surgery if I was not to be crippled by long term pain. I underwent surgery and was told although the outcome of my procedure was successful I could anticipate long term problems as I aged and must expect a level of pain and disability in my later years as surgery could repair but not restore.

I have been performing the Ritual for several years now. I am pain free, mobile and athletic. I am well. I am full of energy. I am full of aspirations and plans for my future years. Would I be like this if I had never begun to perform my Ritual? My spinal surgeon's predictions tell me no.

I know the man I was, the physical and particularly, because it is important, the psychological shape that I was in before my Ritual began. I was preparing to be old. I was booked in for regular health checks. I was sorting out my pension and wondering how my money would 'eke out' if I were to need long term care. I no longer went to work on my building site, (now, I am back on the roof). I was concentrating instead on scaling down my life.

The Ritual has completely altered my perception of the man that I am, the state I am in and the potential that I have. The entire mental exercise of the Ritual takes just over 40 minutes of my day to perform.

It may seem ludicrous, it may seem insubstantial or foolish, but I will repeat until

'I am blue in the face', just give it a go.

Let the Ritual you create, or my Ritual if you are going to replicate my exercises, show you what it can do for your own life.

As you apply therapeutic touch to the area of your body below your fingers be aware of the structures within you under the surface of your torso. Concentrate and mindfully connect with the tissues beneath the skin. Consider the form of your musculature. Imagine the kidney held, supported, and working as efficiently as it has ever done. Create a direct contact through thought between your brain and your kidney functioning. Praise it. Offer your opinion to your kidney that it has never worked more effectively. Be enthusiastic. Connect with your kidney on the right side and then switch hands to the left side of your body and working on the left side repeat this exercise. Perform at least 20 pumping motions on each side of the body in the area of the right and left kidney.

3. THE RITUAL FOR THE PANCREAS

The pancreas is one of the glands forming our endocrine system. It is located in the abdomen. The role of the pancreas is to produce important enzymes to make sure that food is digested and to produce insulin and other hormones to control blood sugar levels. If the pancreas is not in good working order or blocked by a tumour the body is in serious trouble.

Look at the pancreas in an anatomy textbook. It is described as fish shaped but I see it as the shape of a small banana. I work the tissues on the surface of my skin as shown in fig 7.3 and imagine connecting with the pancreas in the position it is tucked in to within the structures within my gut and abdomen. I repeat my Ritual of targeting visualisation by means of therapeutic touch and make my silent affirmations, asserting my pancreas is in great shape and doing a great job.

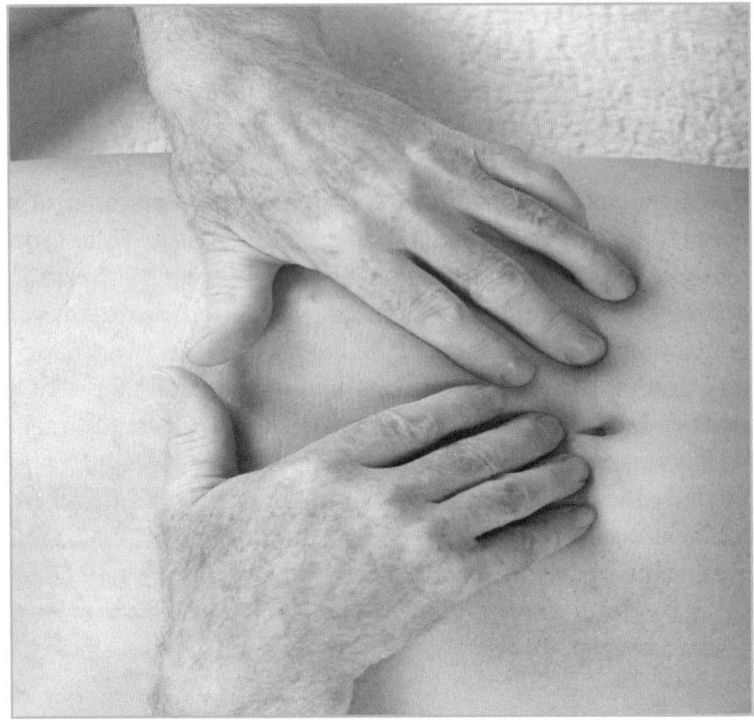

Fig 7.3

I push the fingertips of the left hand gently in to the stomach wall to the left of and one inch above the naval. Pull in the stomach muscles and then release the muscles outwards beneath my fingers creating the sensation that the movement of the surface muscle tissue is being driven by the deepest muscles within myself, coming deep from within the body, from the area around the abdominal cavity.

I see my pancreas as a shiny steel chamber, capsule shaped, releasing a droplet of oil in to my blood stream. I see the oil droplet mix in with the fluids in the pipework of my mechanised body machine and be carried around the engine increasing engine power.

I pump the tissues in the area of the pancreas at least 20 times.

You may wonder why I suggest a repetition of 20 times for each individual exercise?

I felt at least this level of repetition of each exercise was necessary to create the necessary mind body connection between area worked upon and the brain. 10 repetitions were not enough in my case to cut out all other 'noise' and 'chatter' and make the connection required. I found by the time I had performed 20 repetitions of my pumping action I was aware that the focus of my brain was upon the area of my body worked upon. I felt the necessary and powerful mind-body connection had been made. For you the ideal pattern may be to therapeutically pump the tissues in any particular area of the body you are working with only 15 times or to need to work the tissue with my described fingertip massage up to 30 or 50 times. It matters not. If you have the time it is up to you, it is your daily Ritual you are working upon, this is mine.

4. THE RITUAL FOR THE LIVER

The liver sits on the right of the stomach. It is a large rubbery organ protected by the rib cage. We all have some idea of what our liver does as we associate drinking excess alcohol with liver damage!

The liver works to clean up our blood. It filters blood coming from the digestive tract and detoxifies it. When we take drugs our liver bears the impact, metabolising drugs to ensure they work with our body chemistry.

To locate the liver and apply therapeutic touch to the tissue in the area of the liver tuck the fingertips of both hands under the lowest rib bone on the right hand side of the rib cage.

Let your fingertips spread out along the length of the bone. Breathe in as your fingers sink deeper in to the tissues. Create the connection between your brain and the therapeutic touch you are applying. To focus the therapeutic touch delivered upon your liver and direct your mind to apply itself to the task of regeneration and purification of the liver, visualise your liver working.

In the machine of my body I see my liver as a large pink rubbery chamber. I imagine it gurgling and processing engine fluids. I see dirty fluid flowing in to it and clear fluid flowing out. I imagine the engine chamber of the liver full of liquid and then I imagine it emptied. I visualise lifting an inspection hatch and using a steel brush to scrub the inside of the liver chamber, scrubbing out the emptied tank until the inside of it is restored to pink with all the gunk on the walls removed.

I make my silent affirmations, delivering praise and gratitude as I apply therapeutic touch to my skin with my hands positioned as shown in fig 7.4

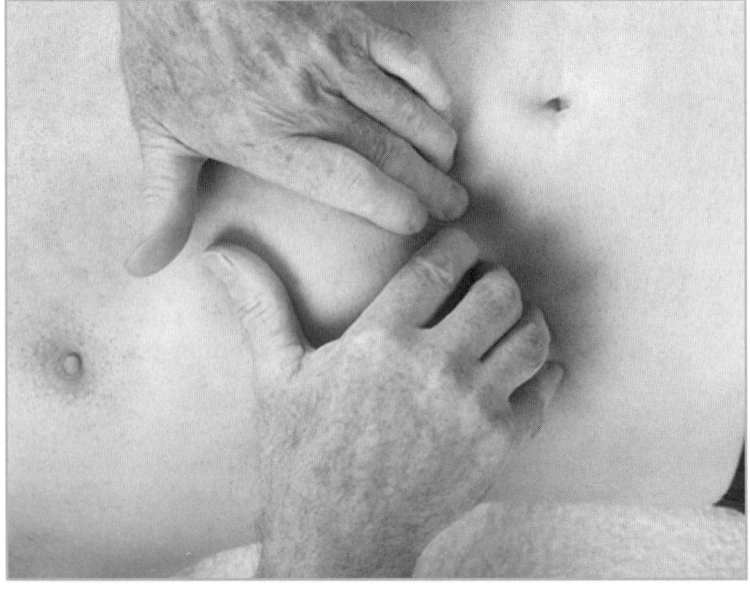

Fig 7.4

You will, I hope at this stage, have come to understand that part of the job of connecting with your inner being is to know what you look like on the inside. Most of us haven't a clue where the major organs of the body are located, what our nervous system looks like or our skeleton.

Mind-body communication depends upon a constant flow of information exchanged between body and mind. For any part of the body to work the brain must direct and co-ordinate action. The effect of the Ritual is that for the duration of your meditative act, in the time taken to apply therapeutic touch, to visualise a particular organ or body part doing a particular job, you take the attention of the brain to the specific act in hand. Effectively in the minutes you perform the Ritual you intervene in the pattern of communication between body and mind, you become orchestrator of your health; for a handful of minutes every day, you become director of your brain.

5. THE RITUAL FOR THE HEART

I now give the heart some attention.

When you engage in the Ritual you engage in practical terms with restoring, maintaining and re-energising the heart, the functional centre of the body you move around in.

When I begin this part of my Ritual I position my right hand. I breathe in forcefully and slowly expel the air I have inhaled. As I exhale I imagine taking hold of my heart and placing it in the centre of my hand. I hold my hand in a claw like shape as this allows me to imagine I am reaching in to myself and taking hold of my heart.

Visualise the heart as a powerful steel pump sitting in the centre of the machine of your being. Imagine it attached to every other cog and wheel in the machine of yourself and imagine it beating. Visualise every metal valve and chamber opening and closing in perfect synchronicity.

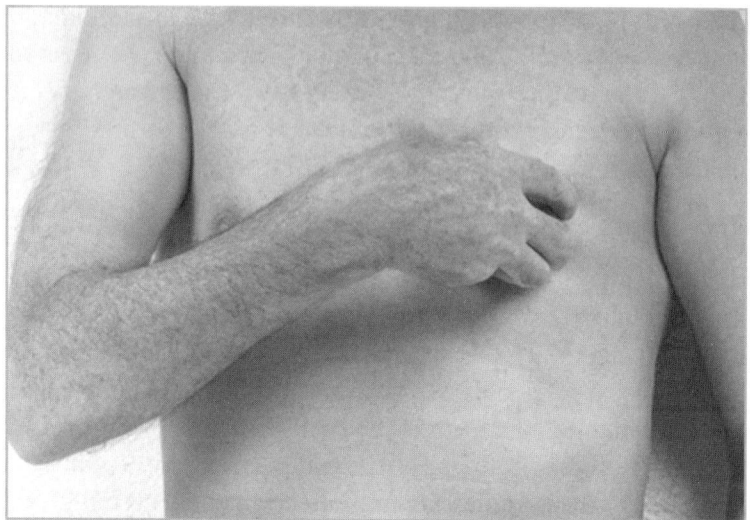

Fig 7.5

As you press in your fingertips to the skin in the area above the heart emotionally connect with the power this organ has. Silently affirm that the job the heart is doing is awesome.

Affirm that the capacity of the heart to pump in the way that it does, is endless.

I visualise a powerful steel pump pumping fluids to every nut, bolt, piston, sensor, plug, axle and cog within the machine of myself.

I focus the power of my mind upon my heart. I affirm how powerful and magnificent my heart is before directing all of my thought compassionately and lovingly to acknowledge the job the pump at the centre of the machine of myself does, each and every day.

Let gratitude ooze through you from your fingertips in to your heart

When I mentally take hold of and fold my hand around my heart at the outset of the exercise I make the connection between heart and mind.

Pressing and releasing my fingertips in to my skin, and flexing the muscles around the chest cavity, is my method of holding the concentration of my brain, of maintaining the link between the processes of the brain and the organ I wish to stimulate.

6. THE RITUAL FOR THE LUNGS

To stimulate the tissues in the area of your lungs it would be most effective to put your hands on your back. It is impossible to do this comfortably and so I place the fingers of the left hand on the side of the right chest cavity as shown in fig 7.6.

My lungs are my powerhouse, receiving my breath and circulating oxygen to every organ, system, and cell in order to maintain my life.

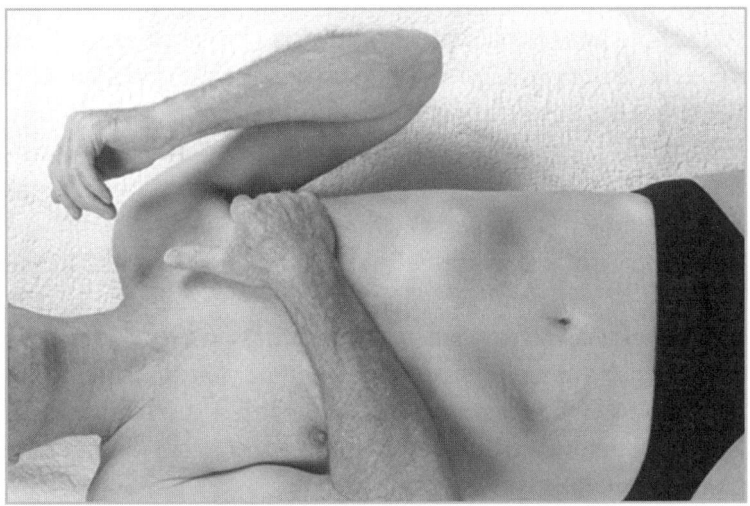

Fig 7.6

I breathe in forcefully, hold each breath and exhale. As I inhale I feel the movement in my ribcage. I visualise a steel box in the engine of myself I open to reveal inside two bellow shaped areas of pink sponge each filled with a thousand air sacks. I see pipes connected to the chamber forcing in air, filling the air sacks and inflating the sponge until it is hardly contained within the steel box. I feel the powerful thrust of air released as the areas of sponge deflate and the increasing power within the air sacks as more air is taken in.

As I work my tissues I marvel at the job my lungs are doing. I observe the perfect sponge structure of my lungs and the thousand air sacks filling and emptying in unison. I recognise the skill involved and give thanks for the job that is done. I have no doubt my lungs are capable of sustaining me. I affirm that my lungs are healthy and clean and powerful and that the job they do is magnificent.

I take 20 breaths in this way, inhaling and exhaling, constantly connecting with the perfect way in which my lungs hold and release air. I would stress I inhale to my fullest capacity and exhale in a slow controlled contemplative way relishing the power of my breath.

I hold gratitude and love in my mind and allow this emotion to flood in to my lung while I work the tissues in the manner shown in the image above.

When I have completed the exercise on my right lung I place my right hand in a similar position on my left chest cavity and work my lungs in a similar way. This time I concentrate my mind on the perfect way in which my left lung is working, giving thanks for the job it is doing. I repeat the same pattern of forced inhalation and exhalation twenty times on the left hand side.

THE PITUITARY SHOWER

This exercise requires reference to a text- book of anatomy. Without a text -book of anatomy I believe almost any one reading this book will be unable to locate the position of the pituitary gland in the brain, let alone visualise it.

The 'Pituitary Shower' is the only Ritual exercise I did not draw from my own imagination.

I was inspired to include a Ritual exercise dedicated to energising my pituitary gland by a technique referred to by Candace Pert, in her wonderful book *Molecules of Emotion.* I give full credit to Candace Pert for introducing me to the idea of the rewards of stimulating the pituitary gland.

The benefits of performing a guided visualisation involving the pituitary gland was suggested to Candace Pert by her friend Evelyn Silvers. The circumstances in which Candace Pert first performed an exercise similar to my christened 'pituitary shower' is recounted in full within the pages I refer to in the *Molecules of Emotion.* (2) Before reading the work of Candace Pert I did not know that the pituitary gland contained the highest concentration of the most potent endorphins the body possesses. I know this now and armed with this knowledge I adapted my Ritual to focus upon it.

I believe the very action of concentrating upon the pituitary gland increases the effectiveness with which the pituitary gland performs. I visualise a small pea sized gland. I place my hands between the outer edges of my eyes and my ear on the top of the cheekbone. I flex the muscles in the roof of my mouth which translates to movement of my skin under my fingers. I visualise stimulating the pituitary gland. I imagine the gland increasing production of all hormones it is responsible for, including human growth hormone, and the hormones and endorphins being showered around the body, almost as if a firework has been lit. The benefits of the hormones and endorphins dispersed seen as a showering of bright sparks throughout my system.

I silently affirm that I am filled with joy, beneficial energy and happiness.

Try it.

It feels amazing.

It is in fact the most amazing exercise in this book.

I cannot describe the benefits, they are not capable of being reduced to words and so I urge any one reading this book to perform this exercise for themselves. I know as I perform this exercise my skeleton, my endocrine system,(3) my nervous system and my immune system benefit. That is the only result I need to cause me to repeat this exercise, day after day after day.

THE END OF EXERCISING; THE BEGINNING OF AWARENESS

This completes the work I do on the principal organs of my body. My Ritual will seem very strange to the uninitiated. To a reader picking up my book and turning casually to this chapter it will seem a performance without sense.

GIVE IT A GO!

BE JOYFUL

BE ENTHUSIASTIC

BE FULLY AWARE OF YOUR OWN POTENTIAL

Something happens. Something it is beyond the power of the words I possess to explain. I continually refer to the consequence of performance of the Ritual as altered life perception. Put more simply, performance of the Ritual has led me to alter the manner in which, I not only see, but connect with ME, the being that I am.

Try it and see what happens.

I suggest it is absolutely impossible to subject the body and mind to the Ritual and maintain old thought patterns, or long held negative opinions about your individual potential and prospects and gifts that you as an individual possess.

Riches will be delivered as your mind set changes. The Ritual leads to changes in health, attitude, performance and well being because it pulls back the sheets and removes the debris and messages of the past to reveal ourselves as we truly are;

an AMAZING work of biological, genetic, and neurological engineering, with unlimited potential.

The only limit upon us is the limit we impose upon ourselves through the thoughts that we carry. The only diseases that can pester us are the ones we harbour and nourish instead of repel. Turn the full force of your energy against what is injuring or ailing you. Turn your whole potential as a magnificent human being towards the rest of your life and see what changes result.

EVERYTHING CHANGES.

BELIEVE IT

And I know you will know within only weeks of a committed performance of the Ritual that you are in control - no one else. Your life is not down to a manager in the NHS or an expensive physician dropping in between ski breaks to pay your body some attention. The shape your future takes, the degree of wellness you possess, the very length of your lifetime, are matters, (setting aside catastrophic and unforseeable events) very much within your gift.

CHAPTER EIGHT

THE EVERY DAY FACE LIFT

Everybody wants to look good but the majority of us do the wrong thing to preserve the looks that we have. I am not talking about smoking cigarettes, drinking too much alcohol, eating foods high in sugars and fats that bloat us and change the image we have. No I am talking about something much more fundamental than that.

I am talking about our ability to do ourselves down, to reduce ourselves, not in the eyes of others, but of ourselves.

One of the most damaging things for our psyche and our appearance is ;

OUR OWN ABILITY TO CRITICISE THE WAY THAT WE LOOK.

When did you last look in the mirror and say something positive to yourself?

Isn't it your habit to say something negative?

' Look at me; I look a wreck?'

'I look pale….grey…sallow…white…red….blotchy…pale…fat!'

When is the last time you looked at yourself in the mirror and said and thought and really believed the words….

'I look great !'

Well let me emphasise this, the first lesson to be learned before you even consider placing your hands in position to start the group of Ritual exercises that make up the everyday facelift is this; if you do not believe you are looking good, that you are glamorous, regardless of the shape of your mouth, size of your nose, length of your eyelashes, nobody else will!

It is not the stereotypically beautiful, (objectively to the masses), 'best looking' people in the room that get the most attention? Have you ever noticed that?

No?

Do you know who it really is?

It is the people who believe in themselves. They are the people to shine.

How do they do that?

Why do those of indifferent looks manage to capture all the attention, exuding a charisma that others simply don't possess?

How can someone with irregular features, even ugliness, (judged by the objective standard of the masses), or a receding hairline come to believe in themself to such an extent that they command a room, drawing everyone around them in?

Simple!

They do naturally what the Ritual is teaching you to do. They regard themselves from another perspective, not the one we automatically impose upon our being, the judgmental, self critical, assessment. They never do that, instead they regard themselves as magnificent, adopting naturally the altered perspective repeated performance of the Ritual will lead you to.

Try it?

Why not, you have come this far, and you have, I presume bought this book with the intention of giving my Ritual a go.

Settle down in the chair that you now use to perform the Ritual or lie down on the bed upon which you perform the Ritual and relax. Breathe deeply and let your mind attain the meditative state the Ritual requires. Sense the physicality of yourself, be aware of the dimensions of your physical body. Create an image in your mind of your body sitting in the chair or lying on a bed. Make the thoughts you direct towards the image of yourself compassionate. Make them loving. Direct this loving and compassionate energy from your mind to the physical mass that you are as you sit or lie as I describe.

If it is too unusual, consider the love you have for your child, your partner, your parent, your spouse, or for a human being you are in love with. Feel the loving energy you create in your emotions for that other person and then turn the emotion on yourself. Let love and compassion flood in to your head and penetrate beneath your skull and behind your eyes. Feel your head fill with the heat of the compassion and tenderness and love directed to your physical body by your thoughts.

How are you feeling?

Look in the mirror.

What do you see?

I bet you see someone you think looks good. Look at the light in your image. Consider the sparkle in your eyes.

I guarantee this is not a moment when you say, ' I look a wreck'. No chance. If you have done as I instructed your image will inevitably be transformed before your eyes.

This exercise never fails.

I have tested it on all of my friends.

Out of it the every day face- lift was born.

People that reach in to their own being and deliver as much love and compassion to the person they find there as they deliver to everyone else cannot help but shine. They cannot help but be magnetic because they are full of a life energy that is rejuvenating. That is accessible to all. More accessible than expensive treatments, face-lifts and anti-ageing creams. The only reason we do not utilise the power we have within us to keep ourselves looking good is I believe because we do not know an everyday face-lift is within our gift or begin to understand the potential we have to slow the body clock of ageing or adjust the movement within its ticking mechanism to retain the energy of our youth.

I certainly did not know and I certainly did not look upon myself with compassion. Twelve years ago I booked myself in for a lower face-lift. This is a one stitch procedure to tighten the neck area. It was disastrous. My surgeon sceptical that any benefit would be achieved advised me against the procedure. I was undergoing the procedure as a prophylactic measure. I was fifty eight. I looked great, my surgeon told me that, but when I looked in the mirror I saw the beginning of age and a slackening of the tissue. I was insistent upon the procedure and I got what my vanity deserved. I looked worse after surgery and I had to cope with significant keloid scarring which develops in rubbery wheals as the tissue grows lumpy and larger than the wound healed.

I spent the next twelve months massaging and connecting with the tissues beneath my fingers and more importantly connecting with the being that I was. I wanted to heal the scarring but in working upon the scars I created a healing regime. Nothing came instantly, for over twelve months the scarring on my face remained much the same but then I noticed changes. The scars were less raised, less obvious, until with constant work they flattened out and resolved. Today it is not evident I underwent this procedure and I know because of the effectiveness of my daily Ritual and the youthfulness it delivers I will never need to undergo surgery again.

The technique I allow you to access through a performance of the Ritual is not rationed, or expensive or only for the few.

Psychologically, because of its universal availability it will seem to have no value, but that could not be further from the truth. Love and compassion directed to the body from the mind makes the body brighter.

I believe our cells are rejuvenated, and I believe that is why my every-day face lift is the only face-lift I need. I was remote and disconnected from myself when I saw plastic surgery as a solution. I am now connected with the physical and mental being that I am. I am in a place of power that delivers what surgery and pills cannot.

HOW MANY OF YOU READING THIS BOOK CAN SAY THE SAME?

If you are still with me, are you willing to create your own daily routine, to give the Ritual a go?

We have arrived at chapter 8. If you are still reading, you understand I presume, something about the power of belief, of persuading the mind of a fact and the impact this belief has upon the body, or in this case, the face you are dealing with.

When we are compassionate towards ourselves, when we direct the mind to deliver love and compassion to our own self, we become not only invincible, we become beautiful. Not just in our own eyes but in the eyes of everyone else. It is at once a mysterious and marvellous fact of our human existence.

The 'everyday face – lift' I describe is about a lot more than turning you in to the best looking man or woman on earth. Only nature can do that. We don't all come with the human beauty stereotype imprinted upon our genes. The stereotypical beauty that registers perfectly with the concept of beauty shared by the majority of our species may never be ours. The every-day facelift does not say that you will be voted Mr Universe or Miss United Kingdom within 28 days of following the Ritual exercises but the Ritual does promise that within a period of weeks of following the programme set out in these pages you will be regarded differently by all around you. In this time period through a daily performance of the Ritual you will have changed the way in which you yourself regard yourself. That is the powerful transition.

Back will come to you the energy and radiance of your youth. It will be you, the faces in the crowded room, turn towards, you, that draws people in. Instead of ageing, withering away in a neglected corner of the room, beset by all the insecurities your life has harboured, you will be circulating!

It is extraordinary but gone will be the need to compare and judge yourself against the supposed dynamism and potential of others. It is your own potential and dynamism you will recognise.

Some people I have met in my life have obviously accessed naturally the technique that I try to guide you to with my Ritual. Some people are so demonstrably ageless, energised and vibrant they will never look old or require an everyday facelift.

The best smile I have ever received in my life was delivered to me by a woman in Cuba with broken teeth and skin like the hide of an elephant.

Do you know what made it so great?

Because, at the moment she smiled, she was radiant. She might have been 106 or she might have been 38. When I regarded her I did not think for one moment of her age.

In the instant she smiled at me my own life was made rich. The smile that came from her struck the very centre of my being. It delivered to me something unforgettable so that now twenty years later I want to write about it.

Through my daily practice of the Ritual I have come to accept there is another dimension to myself, to all of us. I understand ageing is much more complicated than chronological progression. I understand health is much more complicated than pills and consultations. To be the best we can be we cannot rely on a state national health service, we really do have to rely upon ourselves and to do that we have to utilise every gift that we have. Directing our under utilised positive and loving emotion towards ourself really is an appearance changing act

Each of us, every one on this earth represents an amazing piece of art. Our individual sculptures may have very different shapes but the tag attached to each one of them reveals a value beyond gold or any available wealth accumulated on any continent.

Hold that thought and let's begin to make ourselves look the best that we can.

FACIAL TISSUE AND CHEEKBONES BENEATH

As a rule I normally perform manual lymphatic drainage to my neck and face prior to beginning my everyday face lift. (See Chapter 6).

I do this because, after my research for this book, I believe that one of the causative factors in skin ageing is the reduction in the ability of the lymphatic system to remove dead cells and toxins from the cells of the epidermis as we age. I believe the lymphatic system becomes less efficient and more attenuated with age and inevitably benefits from the attention my Ritual gives it.

Having completed my Ritual of stimulating lymphatic drainage in the lymph nodes in my neck and face I continue to dedicate my Ritual exercise to rejuvenating, (I see that as plumping up), the cells of my face.

To begin, relax, place both hands over your face palms down.

Breathe deeply.

Allow your brain to enter in to the state of mindful concentration you will now be familiar with.

Let love and compassion flow through you directing the emotion on to your facial tissues. Feel the warmth of your emotion permeate your skin and reach the cheekbones beneath. With your tissues taut, flex the muscles of your face and imagine rejuvenating fluids pass through the tissues beneath your fingers to the surface of the skin.

Target the positive emotion you create in your mind upon the areas of your face that are most likely to demonstrate signs of ageing, particularly the neck, the tissues around and under the eyes. Focus upon the soft tissues of the cheeks and the lips, paying attention to the area of skin above the top lip.

LEFT SIDE OF FACE AND JAW

Continuing to hold the state of mindful concentration created I begin to apply therapeutic touch to the left hand side of the face. This stimulates lymphatic drainage. The movement of the fingers on the surface of the facial tissues should be hardly perceptible. Pressure applied by the fingertips should gradually increase.

Connect with each area of the surface of the face. Increase the rhythm at which the fingers are pressed in to the facial tissues and released, effectively speeding up the rate at which contact is made between finger tip and skin. Work gently. Maintain the connection between your mind and the areas of facial tissue your fingertips are moving over. Touch each section of facial tissue at least 20 times, applying therapeutic touch downwards along an imaginary line that could be drawn between the upper edge of the left brow and the bottom of the chin on the left hand side

The position of the fingers of my left hand are shown in fig 8.1

Connect with the positive emotions you direct to your self, feel love and compassion pressed in by your fingertips

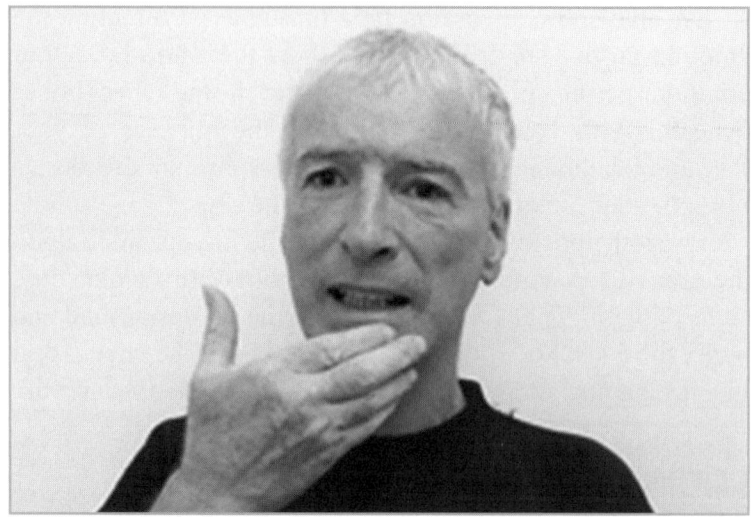

Fig 8.1

to your facial tissue. Visualise your skin tightening under your touch, flex the muscles.

By clenching the jaw as you massage you can elicit a muscle movement beneath the fingertips. Be aware of the message of the positive loving emotion you hold in your mind passing through the deepest of the facial tissues on the left hand side of the face before rising through every layer of facial skin to settle in the surface skin cells. Be mindful of the action you are performing. Imagine the cells under your fingertips plumping up and filling out with the energy of your youth. Imagine lines on the surface of your skin smoothing and disappearing.

RIGHT SIDE OF FACE AND JAW

As shown in Fig 8.1 with hand reversed to opposite side of jaw.

Apply the fingertips of the right hand to the right side of the face. Repeating the technique of application of therapeutic touch to the face as described in the previous exercise move the fingertips downwards, facial section by facial section, from the right brow to the bottom right side of the chin. This is effectively working as lymphatic drainage does.

FACIAL TISSUE BELOW THE EYES

Position your hands as shown in Fig 8.2

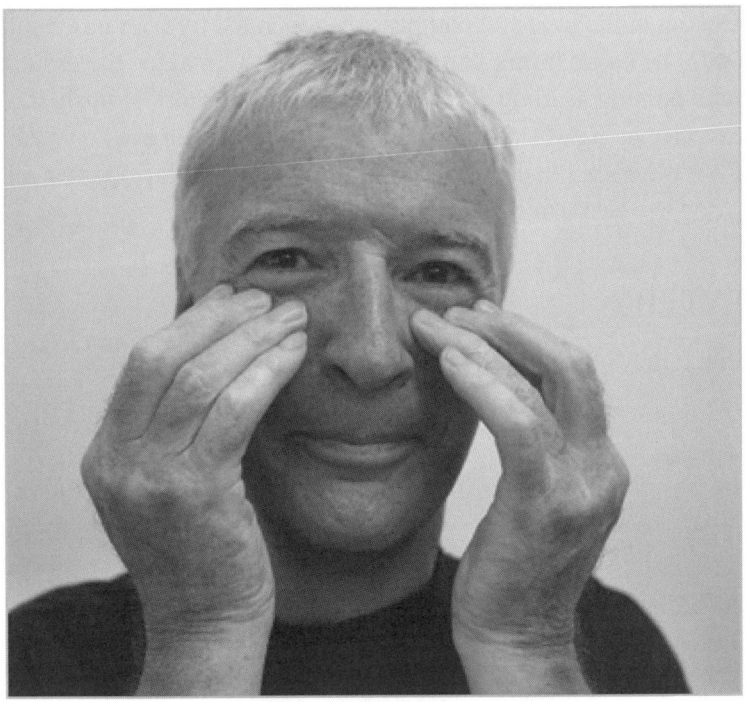

Fig 8.2

Our task with this exercise is to concentrate upon the facial tissue just below the eye. Place three fingertips of the left hand in a horizontal line just below the edge of the bone of the eye socket. Scrunch the cheeks up to obtain movement in the tissues beneath the fingertips. Mentally connect with this movement and with each tightening of the tissue in to a scrunch, draw the energy in the movement to the surface of the skin just beneath the fingertips. A series of 20 short sharp but gentle squeezes of the cheek muscles will produce a discernible movement of the surface of the skin beneath your fingers. Connect with the therapeutic touch you are applying. Concentrate the mind upon the task. Throughout all facial exercises with the Ritual maintain the state of positivity you have created in your mind and direct the love and compassion generated by your emotions on to the tissue layers you are working with. Imagine the tissues rejuvenating firming and plumping as you work. Finish this exercise by lightly stroking the tissue beneath each eye outwards from the corner of each eye to the ear by running the index finger along the curve of the eye socket.

EYELIDS.

Place the fingertips as shown in Fig 8.3

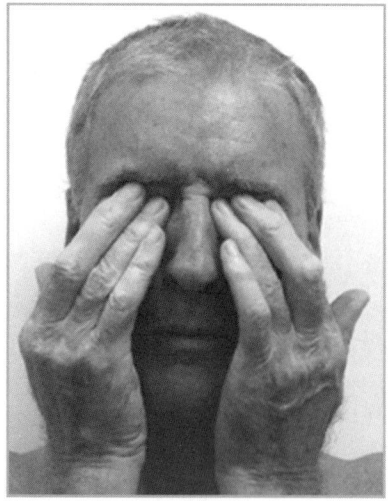

Fig 8.3

Maintain the state of mindful concentration created and hold the positive loving and compassionate emotion generated in your mind. Turn the attention of your mind to the outer edge of the eyelids, to the area vulnerable to the development of deep lines we so charitably describe as, 'crows feet'.

Place hands as shown in Fig 8.3

Place the fingertips of the left and right hand in the position shown and again scrunch up the cheek muscles sensing the movement in the tissue under the fingertips. Draw the energy of this movement up through the basal layers of facial tissue and sense the energy beneath your fingertips. Visualise your face without lines beside the eyes, visualise your skin smoothing as you work.

Tighten and relax the cheek muscles on each side of the face, beside the corner of each eye at least 20 times.

Relax.

I think it important that I make a point that should be borne in mind as each facial exercise is performed and indeed to performance of every exercise within the Ritual.

As you apply therapeutic massage to the tissues of the face it is important that you believe in the efficacy of your actions. We have to believe the exercise performed is having a beneficial effect upon the cellular structure of our cells and believe that flooding the tissue with positive attention can and is delivering therapeutic consequences.

If you believe the massage you perform is straightening out dryness, tiredness, fine and even deep lines to restore the energy you had and the glow you possessed twenty or even thirty years ago your Ritual will be effective. Don't ask me how, but it will. It will not wind you back to the age of 35, you will not look in the mirror and see yourself within minutes of Ritual exercising as you were then but you will see a youthful fresher man or woman looking straight back at you out of the mirror.

The Ritual is about retrieving lost energy, vigour.

When we are in love we look years younger, have a spring in our step, give the impression to all around us of being on mood altering drugs or to have stepped out of a health farm when of course we have taken no action at all save to change the emotion our brain generates. Love is a powerful emotion, even when it is directed upon other beings, it has the power within it to make the one bestowing love look better. The Everyday Facelift teaches us to harness the benefit of loving and compassionate energy and to direct it upon ourselves to obtain the same results. Through focus and mindful concentration it is possible to direct the most positive of emotions upon our own cells. This does not deny any one the gift of loving well, as many people in their life as they can, it simply allows an unusual turn of events, the transformative action of loving ourselves in a similar and astonishingly rejuvenating way.

CHEEKS

Place hands as shown in Fig 8.4

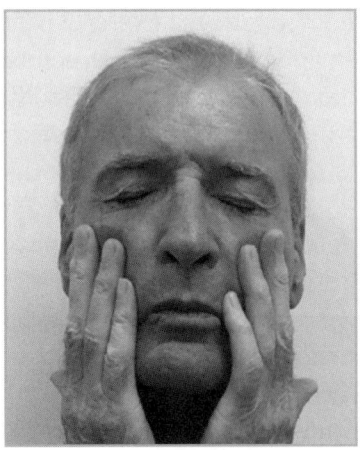

Fig 8.4

Place the hands palms downwards on to the cheeks.

Remain in state of mindful concentration. Direct loving and compassionate thought as you apply therapeutic touch to the cheeks. Our work is to plump and firm the tissues in the area of our cheek- bone, to help define the bone.

Position your hands as shown. The highest part of the left cheek should be covered with the fingertips of the left hand. Scrunch up the facial muscles in the cheek. Feel the tissues under your fingertips move. Connect with the energy of this movement. Visualise the cells in the tissue of the cheeks plumping up. Imagine each cell within the tissue filling with the energy of your youth as you work upon it. Flood each cell within the structure of your cheek, with the loving and compassionate emotions you are holding within your mind. Imagine the tissue receiving this emotion gratefully and renewing itself. Tighten and relax each cheek 20 times. On each flex of your facial muscles pull the energy of the movement up through the deepest layers of facial tissue to the surface of each cheek.

FOREHEAD

Place hands as shown in Fig 8.5

The fingers of each hand should be flat against the skin of the forehead.

Remaining in a state of mindful concentration and holding the emotion of love and compassion flex the muscles in the forehead. I put an exaggerated expression of surprise upon my face.

Register the movement of the skin of the forehead beneath your fingertips. Focus upon it while directing the full energy of your thought to the forehead. Visualise the skin softening and tightening. Imagine lines upon your brow erased.

Flex and release the muscles of the forehead 20 times.

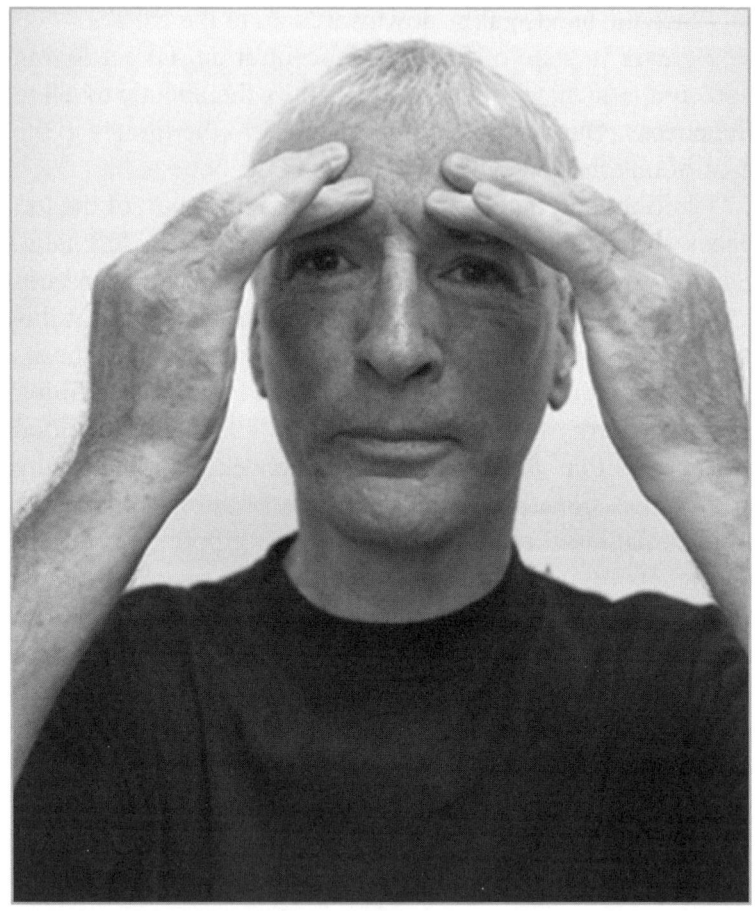

Fig 8.5

LIPS

I perform three Ritual exercises for the lips.

I work on the area above the top lip. I work on the top lip itself and I work on the bottom lip. The position of my fingers is shown in Fig 8.6 –Fig 8.8

Place the fingertips as shown in Fig 8.6

AREA ABOVE THE TOP LIP

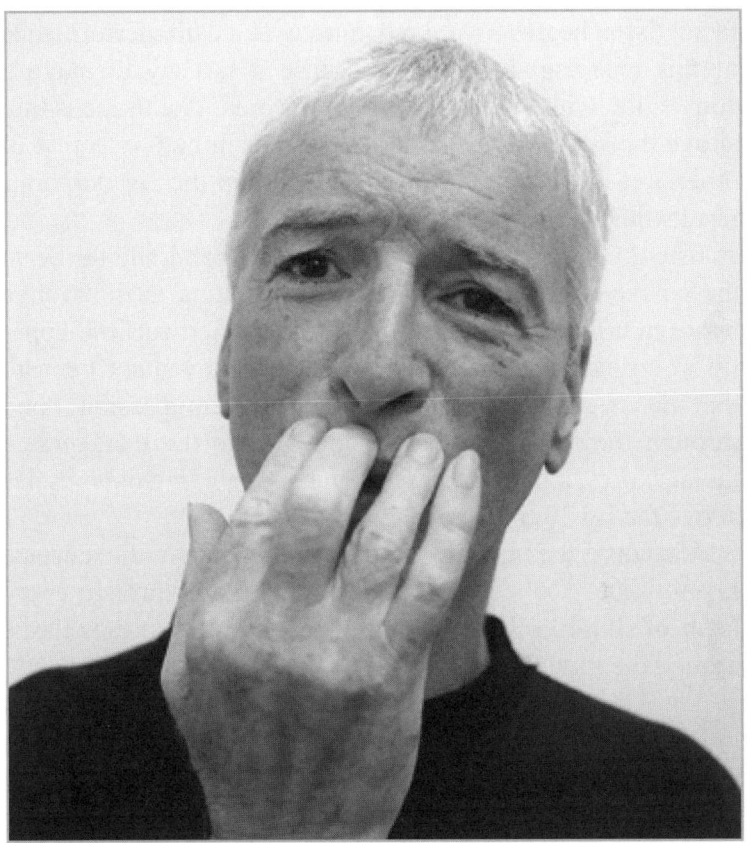

Fig 8.6

The area above the lips needs a lot of work, which means it needs a lot of positive mind energy compassion and love directed upon it. Women are particularly sensitive about the lines and furrows that appear above the top lip but men are not immune. The change in the structure of the tissues above the top lip and a narrowing of the lips is one of nature's most demonstrable insults. An open faced joyous freshness is difficult to maintain when the mouth is tightly drawn. It is therefore remarkable to observe how swiftly this area of facial tissue begins to look younger with a daily performance of this exercise. It may be because it is easy to make a connection with the tissues within the area. The tissue is thin above the lips and lip tissue is different in nature to that of other areas of the face which may explain the very obvious results the exercise delivers.

The 1st 2nd and 3rd fingers of the left hand should be in the position shown with the 2nd finger resting in the groove between upper lip and nose. Part the lips and curl the upper lip in an exaggerated fashion. Feel the movement beneath the fingertips. Feel positivity love and compassion flood through the fingertips to the skin. Create the exaggerated facial expression formed by tensing and relaxing the muscles above the lip 20 times.

Visualise the movement of collagen from the deepest facial tissue. Feel collagen flowing and rising through every layer of skin to fill and plump the cells in the surface tissue around the mouth.

Place the fingertips in position on the top lip itself as shown in Fig 8.8. Repeat the exercise. Place the fingertips in position on the lower lip as shown in Fig 8.7 and repeat the exercise, pouting and relaxing the lips as you work. As with all of the other exercises, visualise the cells within the lip structure swelling and plumping out as they are filled with the love and compassion directed within each cell from the brain.

THE BOTTOM LIP

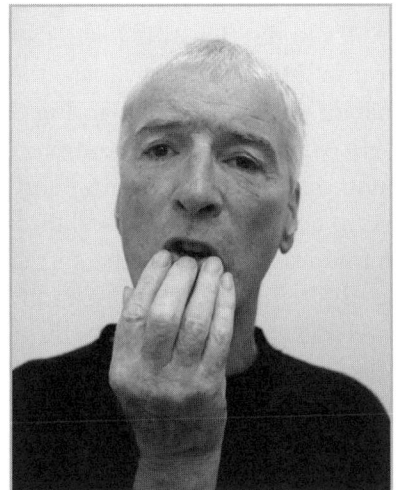

Fig 8.7

THE TOP LIP

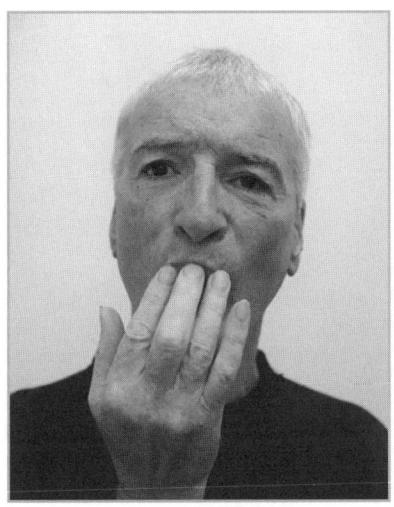

Fig 8.8

NECK AND THROAT

To conclude my Everyday Facelift I work on the tissues of my neck and of my throat.

I place my hands as I demonstrate in Fig 8.9

I hold my state of mindful concentration.

I feel, hold and direct positive loving and compassionate emotion to the skin cells of my neck and throat.

As I work in this way I visualise the surface tissues of my skin responding, tightening, smoothing and filling out.

With my fingertips in position on my throat I contract the muscles in my neck. This allows me to feel movement in the tissues at the side of my throat.

As the muscles in this area flex and contract press the fingertips in to the tissues of the neck 20 times using light pressure.

Move to the nape of the neck and repeat the exercise.

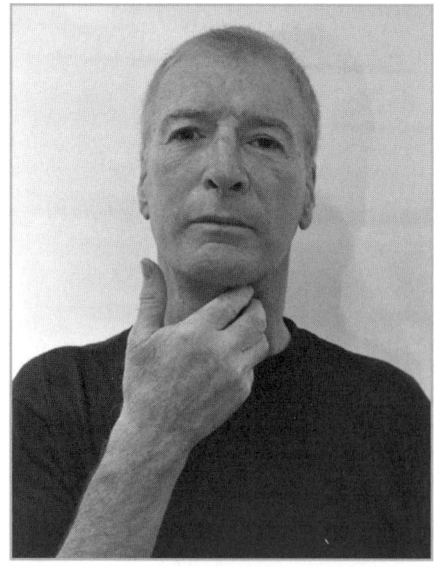

Fig 8.9

SOME OBSERVATIONS

At first, to the beginner, the Everyday Facelift may seem long and complicated, it is not. When you are relaxed, with the necessary mind set as described, the whole procedure need only take a few minutes.

Remember what you have read elsewhere in this book and realise that to perfect a meditative technique, to work with the power of the mind and to realise the benefits of mind-body therapies takes time. Throughout the chapters in which I present my Ritual I refer repeatedly to my state of mindful concentration. It is, as I have said, not a state that is entered naturally at first. The important thing to do is to relax in to it. Consider it unimportant. Simply close your eyes breathe deeply and bring yourself within the skin of yourself. A deep connection must be forged between body and mind if the Ritual is to work.

The state of mind the Ritual requires may be a novelty in your life. I appreciate you may never have concentrated upon drawing your attention inwards. Changing the perspective you have, of the body you have, will deliver results but at first you may find the programme will frustrate you or promote rage and draw derision as you fail to make the connection necessary for the mind to do its work upon the body you possess.

Do not give in.

The Ritual becomes easier with practice. Indeed it becomes addictive, to the point that a day feels incomplete if a Ritual session is missed. The act of repetition of the exercises over a period of time, results in the phenomenon of conditioning. The brain is conditioned to believe. Moving from doubt to a conviction that the face is looking good, delivers the required result.

Conditioning is the gift of every group of exercises within the Ritual. The Ritual causes the brain to rewire, to take our old beliefs, however limiting and debilitating they may be, and consign them to history. As we perform our daily Ritual we slowly create new beliefs, new circuits and links across synapses in our brain, that can have positive and dramatic effects upon our mind and our body.

And the good news is, even if you stall and flounder with your first attempts at performing the facelift described the very physicality of the Ritual facial exercises and the flexing of facial muscles the Everyday Facelift demands will have a toning effect. So hang in there, youthfulness may take a little longer to arrive but firmer looking skin is right there waiting for you, under your fingertips.

One final thought, and one I think it is very important to remember. We cannot all be as chiselled as Hollywood requires but we can all be beautiful.

—————— CHAPTER NINE ——————

THE RECUMBENT GYM AND OTHER MATTERS

THE RECUMBENT GYM

Do you go to the gym or do you stay at home and perform the Ritual?

Before you make a decision remember those athletes in Chapter 4!

After an eight week period in the gym those who put in the physical effort were rewarded with a very noticeable 28% increase in the tone and shape of their thigh muscles. Impressive I agree and it would undoubtedly be worth getting out the car, and making the journey to the gym, and enrolling in a gold membership programme if it were not for the fact that those non-athletes, the stay at home potatoes on the couch, the *visualisers* in the control group, told to simply imagine themselves performing gym exercises, attained a 24% increase in the development tone and shape of thigh muscle. They did it not by working out but by planting a visual image in their mind of the muscles in their thigh developing.

Now that to me is more than impressive. It is impressive and exciting because it is tangible proof of the amazing results that can be attained by turning our attention within ourselves to harness the power of our mind.

Of course some may say there is more pleasure to be had by going to a gym; the camaraderie and competitiveness of the work out, the stimulation of being coached and pushed to the limits by a personal trainer. The gym experience is undeniably different and I do not seek to dissuade anyone from enjoying what their gym provides I simply make the point that the Ritual can achieve the same results or almost the same. Utilising the power you have in your mind, can, as remarkable as it may seem, keep your body in good shape.

Before we start the Ritual exercises for your musculature, I am going to read your mind. I know by now you will have studied the photographs. It is probably the first thing you did on opening this book. How do I know? Because it is what we all do, we, collectively, the readers of the world, in any book with pictures, we consider the pictures first. So I wish to say this. Having looked at the pictures of my physique you may think, he does not look like Ryan Gosling or Bradley Cooper or any 'hunk' that works out. What is he talking about?

I respond by saying this. I am not interested in creating a muscle bound torso. For one thing, all those muscles take a lot of carrying around and each extra pumped up pound adds to strain placed on the joints. I am interested in health and tone. I am interested in elimination of fat.

It does not follow that because you are rippling with muscle you are a powerful gifted or a supreme athlete. Think of Sir Bradley Wiggins, Mo Farah, Peter Crouch. Lithe, stringy, lean, fit, taut. They are the adjectives you would throw at this group of sporting heroes. I am not aiming at big. I am aiming at healthy. I am aiming at the form of longevity and agelessness. At 105 I do not want to be big and mighty and lumbering with knees and hips destroyed from carrying my mass, I want to be spry and nimble and fit as I was twenty five years before.

Lecture over. Let me take you through my mind body work out.

With the recumbent gym I target three areas of my body.

I do not perform a full body work out but you get the point? If you had the time the Ritual would work for you by developing muscle tone and redefining your shape in any area of the body to which it was applied.

The following exercises are basically to tone the muscles of the chest, arms and stomach.

THE PECTORAL MUSCLES

It will now be tedious to repeat the mind should be in a state of mindful concentration at the point each exercise is begun. A mental image should be formed of the body part worked upon which assists the mind with the job it has to do. Either imagine the muscles as powerful steel wires or cords in the machine that you are or lift an image of perfect pectoral muscles from the anatomy textbook.

Hold the image generated and silently affirm the fantastic shape the muscles of your body are in, the amazing job they are doing. Feel gratitude flow from the mind to the muscle group that is targeted and feel the positive emotion of gratitude

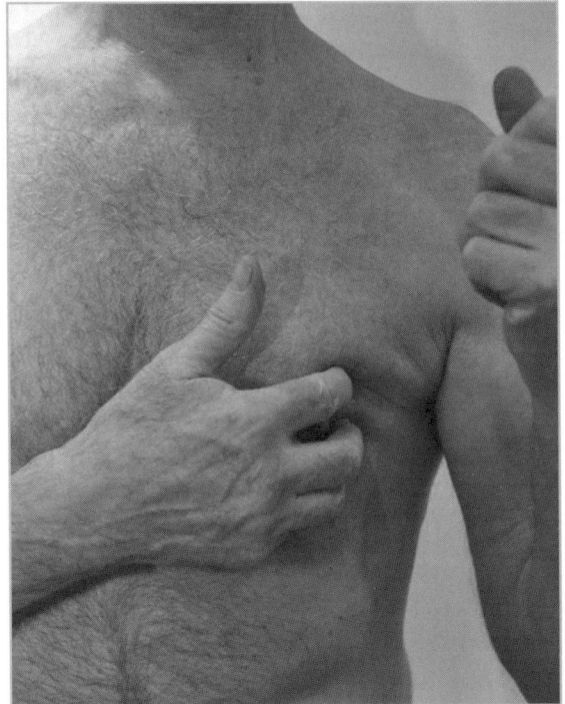

Fig 9.1

and love filling each muscle held. With my right hand in the
position shown in Fig 9.1 with the fingers spread out along
the pectoral muscles, I flex the muscles in my shoulder, arm
and chest which creates movement in the pectoral muscles
my Ritual is targeting. I focus upon this movement as I flex
and relax the muscles in this area. Initially flexing may cause
only a limited amount of movement, but movement achieved
will increase as this muscle group develops. With each slow
flex I visualise the muscle fibres under my fingers swelling
and becoming more powerful. I silently affirm that every
muscle is amazing and doing an amazing job. I repeat the
action described 20 times.

THE ROTATOR CUFF

I position my hands as shown in Fig 9.2

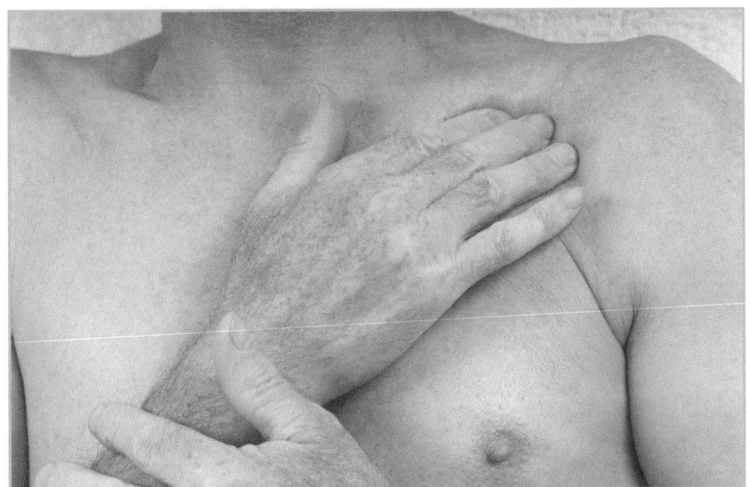

Fig 9.2

The rotator cuff is the group of muscles and tendons that act to stabilise the shoulder. The area of tissue around the rotator cuff of the shoulder appears hollowed out with advancing years. This exercise maintains and firms the muscles in the rotator cuff group.

With the fingers positioned as in Fig 9.2 I squeeze the muscles in the area of the shoulder which produces movement under my fingers. I focus my mind upon this movement. With each slow flex I visualise the muscle fibres as steel cords tightening and swelling and becoming more powerful. I affirm the brilliance of the job the muscles at the shoulder do and will continue to do.

I repeat the action of flexing and relaxing this muscle group 20 times.

THE SHOULDERS
I position my hands as shown in Fig 9.3

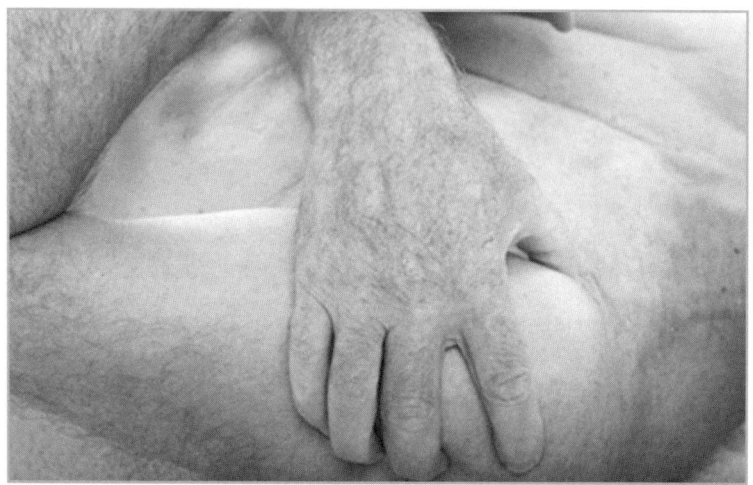

Fig 9.3

Using meditation, visualisation and affirmation I wrap my right hand around my left shoulder as shown. I flex the shoulder muscles. I feel the muscles move under my fingers. My mind is focused upon the task of developing muscle tissue. I visualise the cells in the muscle under my fingers responding and swelling and strengthening as I hold the muscle in a tight grip allowing the whole focus of the positivity and emotion I hold in my mind to be directed within this muscle group. I silently affirm how amazing the muscles under my fingers are and the brilliant job they are doing.

I flex and release the group of muscles in the shoulder 20 times before changing the position of my hands to place my left hand around my right shoulder. I repeat the exercise, working the muscles in my right shoulder in the same way, flexing and relaxing the muscle group 20 times.

THE BICEPS

I position my hand as shown in Fig 9.4

The bicep muscle defines the male. It is the muscle that is flexed to demonstrate prowess and I find the bicep muscles exceptionally responsive to the power within the Ritual.

I place my fingers as shown, and work in the same way I describe in the exercises above, visualising muscle tone, affirming the power within my bicep muscle as I work

I visualise energy being pulled from deep within the muscle to the muscle surface.

I massage the muscle pressing my fingers on to the surface of my skin as the muscle is flexed at least 20 times and I then release the pressure.

With each flex I silently affirm how amazing the muscles are.

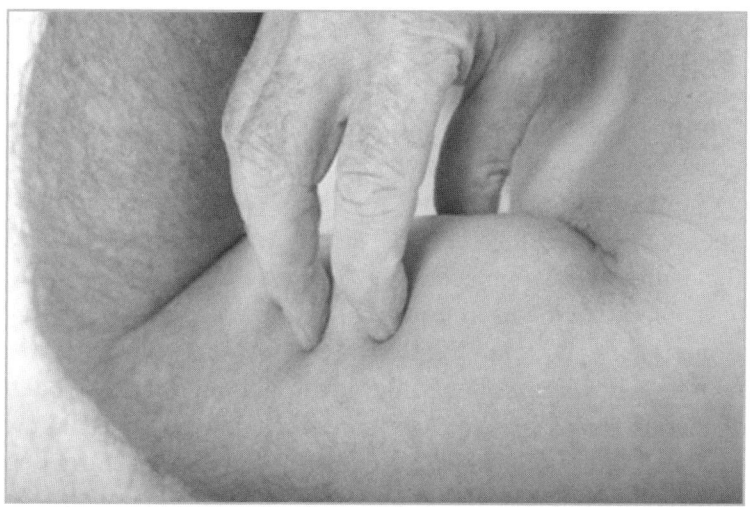

Fig 9.4

The consequence of performing the exercises above is more than simply cosmetic. I not only appear more toned, I am stronger, I can lift greater weights. I can work for longer on manual tasks such as gardening and DIY without tiredness. I think it is important that I state this to be the case. It demonstrates to me the benefits I derive from Ritual exercising are not simply within my mind. I remember when considering the academic literature about the benefits asthmatics achieved in terms of increased lung function, in trials of placebo respiratory medicines, that reports of improved lung function were not objectively verified. The improvement was said to be in the mind of the patient only. I have been impressed that the consequence for me, of my Ritual exercising, is demonstrable in terms of the energy I have which I demonstrate when performing practical tasks. The gains in development of muscle and tone cannot only be in my mind because every day the consequence of my increased and developed musculature is practically demonstrated.

THE ABDOMEN

This exercise needs to be performed lying flat on a bed or on the floor.

I work three different muscle groupings within the abdomen to develop the musculature at the top bottom and the centre of the stomach.

I work first on my lower abdomen positioning my fingertips as shown in Fig 9.5

To work the muscles in the lower abdomen I lie flat and then raise my head and shoulders off the bed just a few inches. I feel the muscles at the base of my stomach tighten beneath my fingertips. My body is in the position it would be in if I was at the gym performing a trunk curl. A trunk curl performed in this way is less stressful for the spine than a conventional sit up. My Ritual trunk curl is enhanced by my visualisation of my muscles tightening and strengthening, my affirmation of their brilliance and my ability to direct the

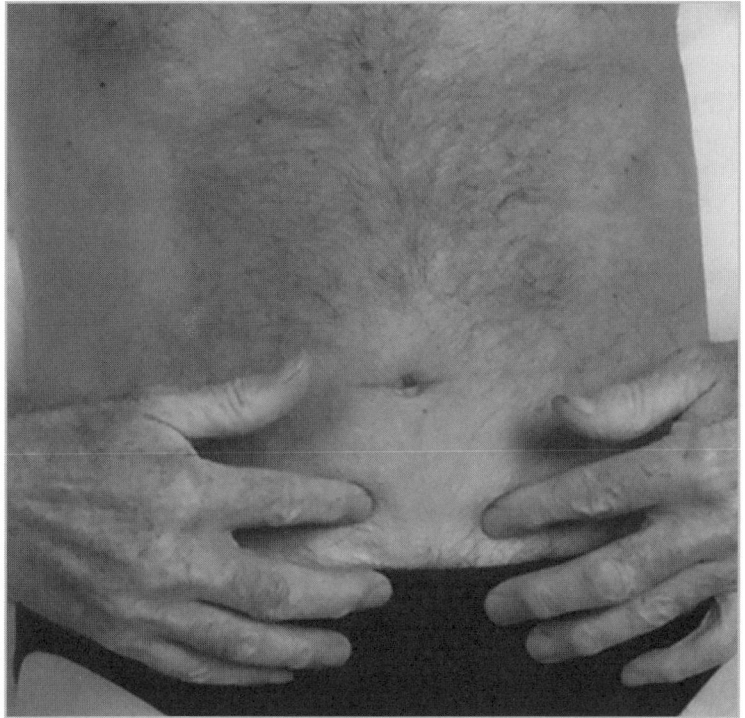

Fig 9.5

full attention of my mind to the task of building muscle by using therapeutic touch. I silently affirm the brilliance of my lower stomach muscles and the marvelous job they are doing to hold and contain me.

I repeat the action of flexing and releasing this muscle group 10 times. As muscles build this number can be increased to 20.

I move my hands upwards to the centre of the abdomen and concentrating on this central muscle group under my fingertips I repeat the exercise.

I move my hands to the top of my abdomen and repeat the exercise for a third time, working on the muscle group at the top of the abdomen'.

A RITUAL FOR MEN ONLY
THE PENIS AND THE PROSTATE

If you worry that you do not have the urinary flow that you used to have twenty years ago or that you may not be able to sustain an erection for as long as you did in your youth, worry no more. The Ritual can I believe help, not only psychologically, but also by delivering physical results.

The Ritual enhances libido, aids sexual performance, improves urinary flow and I believe helps to protect my prostate from the risk of cancer.

Now you may want photographs so that you may follow the movements I describe, and while I do not wish to disappoint, I have to confess that this is the one area of my Ritual I did not wish to pose for.

Nevertheless the exercise is simple to describe and the results of working as I suggest impressive.

The exercise I perform is a variation on a pelvic floor exercise which over decades has been effective in tightening pelvic muscles with consequent benefits for libido and erectile function.

To perform this exercise I place the 1st 2nd and 3rd finger of the left hand in the area between the scrotum and the anus. Flex and tighten the muscles in this area. Tighten the buttocks. Visualise urinary flow increasing with each flex of this muscle group. Visualise a powerful flow of urine running as if a tap had been turned on. Imagine the force of the flow and the bladder as a rubber chamber emptying.

Flex and release the muscles in this area 20 times.

PROTECTING THE PROSTATE.

Locate the bone just above the base of the penis. The sym - physis pubis joint. Place the fingertips of both hands in the soft tissue on the top edge of this bone as shown in Fig 9.6

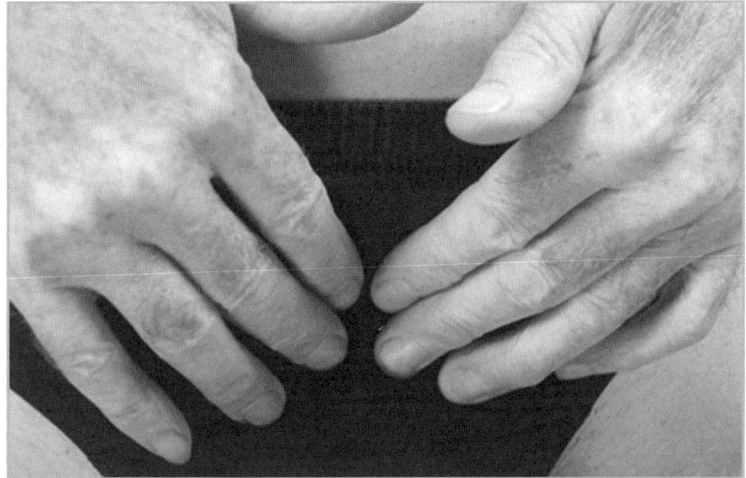

Fig 9.6

Pull the stomach in and let the fingertips sink in to the tissue while pushing the stomach out and make yourself aware of the tissue beneath your fingers and then hold in your mind the sensation of the muscular action in this area. Think of the layers of tissue beneath your fingertips.

Take your mind beneath each tissue layer, deeper and deeper, in to the centre of your being. Connect with the dimensions of yourself. The distance and spaces within you, the distance between the bone your fingertips are placed on and your anus. Consider the fluids and musculature between the two. Consider your penis and testes and the glands that form your reproductive system. Feel the energy that connects your massage to your anatomy and to your brain in one circuit of activity and exchange.

Make your mind concentrate on your prostate gland.

If you fear the gland may be enlarged imagine a hazel nut swollen to the size of a golf ball and visualise with every movement of your fingers the nut shrinking back as the therapeutic massage is delivered. Concentrate on your act of restoring your virility and protecting your prostate from disease. Be mindful of the association between the Ritual and the health of your prostate. Persuade yourself of the connection between your therapeutic massage and increased vigour, renewed virility and enhanced and restored libido. Remember in the Ritual brainwashing is allowed! As with every other exercise perform the therapeutic action of pressing and releasing the fingertips from the tissues beneath them at least twenty times.

All through this exercise continually affirm to the prostate the amazing and healthy state it is in.

ERECTILE DYSFUNCTION

I believe the exercise for the penis and the prostate changes blood supply to the penis. I believe erectile dysfunction can be rectified by changing the nature of messages that are communicated from the mind to the penis. It is absolutely necessary to believe the mind and the body working together can cure any sexual dysfunction that has arisen. It is absolutely necessary to believe that performing the exercise described will restore virility and sexual function. The act of mindful engagement with the penis and the prostate, (the gland producing semen), will result in an improvement of blood supply to the penis.

Belief in the relevance of the exercise to curing any problems of erectile dysfuntion will eventually condition the mind to understand the exercise as performed is the solution to problems which have been experienced. This shift in focus will develop psychological benefits to any male failing to sustain an erection and this psychological shift will of itself improve the situation restoring an expectation of virility, with expectation producing the desired result!

AN EXERCISE FOR BALDNESS

Over twenty years ago I was mortified when during a car journey my niece who was sitting behind me said, ' Uncle Glyn do you know you are going bald?'.

I checked my scalp when I got home and there was undoubtedly thinning hair and a very evident balding patch on my scalp. If nature had been allowed to take its course; if I had accepted like a good percentage of males that I was to face baldness and had grown accustomed to the idea I would in all probability now be totally bald.

When I began the Ritual my hair was thin and patchy on the crown of my head. I wondered if my Ritual if targeted to the area may have an effect upon the speed at which my hair was thinning and the rate at which my hair follicles were succumbing to the natural process of ageing.

I created the following exercise as a prophylactic for my scalp in order to stimulate and rejuvenate the hair follicles in the two areas of the head most prone to balding, the front hair line and the crown of the head.

I am pleased to announce my daily performance has been worthwhile. Not only has my niece's prediction failed to come true, my hair has decided to stop falling out and indeed at the crown has grown back. I now have more hair on my head than I had ten years ago and the hair that I have is thick not brittle and dried out. My hair is grey, but that is not the point. My hair was grey at 35. The point for me is that hair loss has completely stopped and even more miraculously has been reversed.

AN EXERCISE FOR THE BALDING TEMPLES

Place the left fingertips on the front hairline as shown in Fig 9.7

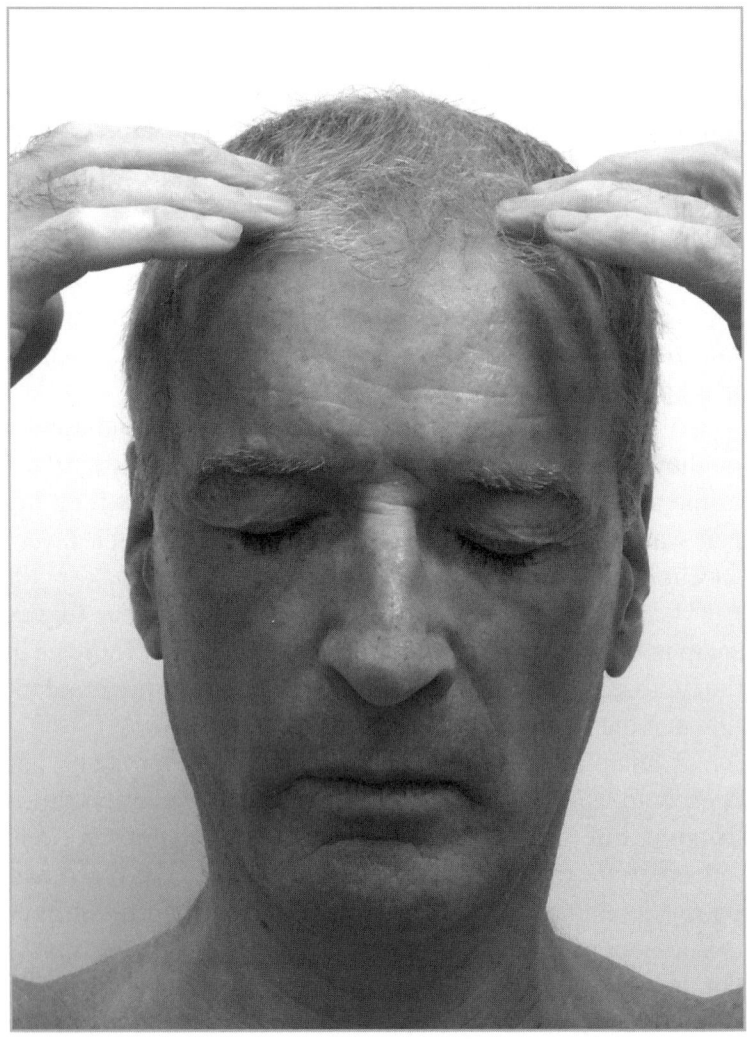

Fig 9.7

With all the Ritual exercises for creating hair growth I place the fingertips of both hands on the scalp in the area I wish to deal with. I create movement in the tissues under my fingers by flexing the muscles in my jaw and mouth. With practice, flexing and releasing the jaw muscles creates movement in the skin over the skull. I sense this movement under my fingers and connect with it. With each flex of skin I visualise hair being pulled through the surface of my scalp and I affirm how amazingly productive my hair follicles are.

I direct the positive emotions of love, compassion and gratitude in to the hairline. I massage the hairline using the little finger of the left hand. Imagine the hairline of your youth. Imagine your hair thick and lustrous growing at speed. Visualise yourself at the barbers. See your hair being cut, raised up at the front hairline by the barbers comb, cut and falling to the ground. Visualise your hair growing once more at the hairline and once more being cut. Hold this imagery. Connect with the positive emotion flooding in to the scalp under your fingertips. Visualise every hair follicle filling with positivity love and compassion. Visualise rows of hair follicles waking up, and returning to work. Apply therapeutic touch to the entire length of the hair line before repositioning your hands upon the crown of the head.

THE CROWN

Place both hands upon the crown of the head, palms down as shown in Fig 9.8

I repeat the exercise I have performed for the front hairline but during this exercise my hands are aligned on my crown with the fingertips positioned on the part of the crown known as the lambdoid suture. I apply my therapeutic massage to the crown continuing from the lambdoid suture to the sagittal suture. In this exercise I think it is important to concentrate

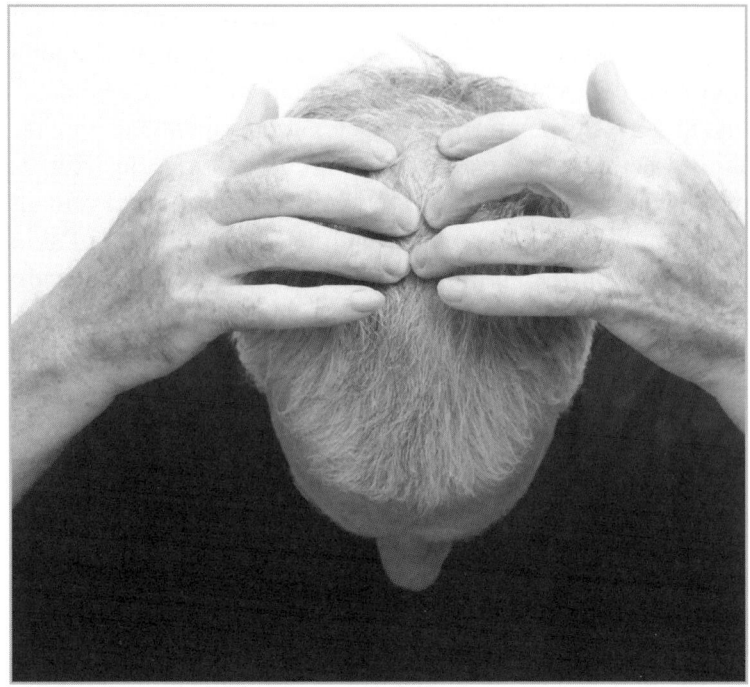

Fig 9.8

on drawing energy upwards from beneath the surface of the scalp in to the hair follicles. I believe this reinvigorates and regenerates biological pathways that may have atrophied with age.

THE RITUAL FOR SPORTING INJURIES

The gift of the Ritual is that I do not feel inclined to give up my pursuit of extreme sports.

My Ritual has taught me,
WE DO NOT HAVE TO BE LIMITED BY THE
CHRONOLOGY OF OUR YEARS
BELIEVE IT

IT IS A FACT
LET THE THOUGHTS YOU HOLD IN YOUR MIND
REJUVENATE YOUR LIFE

One practical consequence of my continued enthusiasm for adventure is the occasional injury.

The Ritual has not turned me in to a super hero. I do still sustain scrapes and knocks which injure me, it is just that now, several years in to my Ritual performance I deal with injury in a different way.

I list here the physical knocks I have suffered over the last few years that I have set my Ritual to work on.

There was no logical point for me in creating a Ritual and setting aside time every day to apply myself to it if when I suffered a sporting injury I booked in immediately for physiotherapy. Indeed physiotherapy would not work for me because I do not believe in it. In fact on the only occasions I have received physiotherapy my pain and disability has been so much worse after a physiotherapy session I have felt as if I have been mugged. Not that I do not say to all those sportsmen satisfied with the physiotherapy they have received that they should not continue to believe in it and indeed book extra sessions. My research for this book demonstrates one evident thing to me about treatments and cures.

IF YOU BELIEVE IN THE CURE DELIVERED IT WILL WORK.

I know also it is the mind working rather than the proposed cure that cures with the cure being the necessary trigger to spur healing, just as my Ritual is the trigger which has on more than one occasion set my mind to work to repair the damage to my body, my enthusiasm for sport has caused.

I list the sporting injuries I have to date worked upon and the results achieved.

MOUNTAIN BIKING

Do not jerk your bike sharply to the left and steer yourself over a one in one slope just to keep up with your mate; certainly not if the route you project your bike and yourself at is a mess of bracken and twisted tree roots. I did just as I describe and when my front tyre snagged in the fork of a root I was projected with such suddenness from my bike seat my legs went over my head curling the whole of my spine before I landed on my neck. I cannot imagine the technicalities of the impact upon the vertebrae at the top of my back or the extent to which every nerve and joint in the area was jarred and ripped. I was numb. I lay on the ground and dare not try to move as I thought I was paralysed. Funnily enough at the time of the accident I did not feel any pain but I did every day afterwards. When I tried to rotate my neck or bend my chin downwards the pain at first was extreme.

I suffered this injury when my Ritual was in its inception. I did not consider the Ritual I was building if applied to my neck could fix any damage sustained. For me initially the Ritual was a preventive therapy. An energy boost I delivered to myself.

As I did not see the Ritual as a tool to deal with injury I went to my GP. I sat through my ten minute consultation and was referred for an X-ray. I sat in the X-ray department of my local hospital, and returned to my GP who announced my X-ray results showed the vertebrae in my neck were damaged through 'wear and tear'; a consequence of my age. The blow from the fall from my mountain bike had set off symptoms I would have experienced in any event without a fall from my bike but which may not have been evident for 10 or 15 years. There was nothing to be done. I was told my neck would always be painful. I was to manage pain relief with paracetamol and ibuprofen and give up mountain biking!

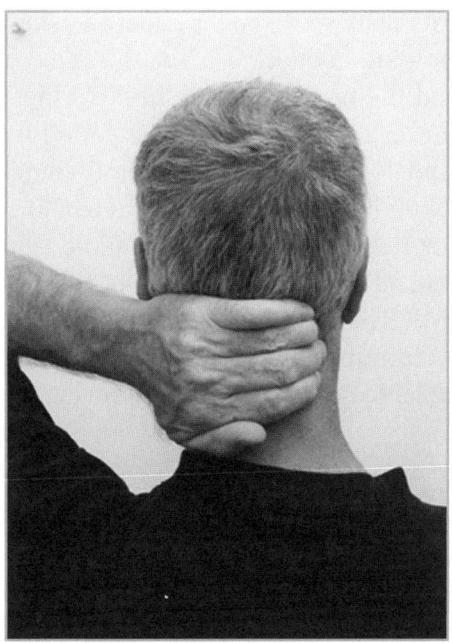

Fig 9.9

I did as advised and the pain gradually subsided but did not go away. Over the next few years I was aware of my old injury. From time to time pain in my neck flared and I would suffer stiffness and restricted movement all over again. Eventually, disillusioned and in a state of some desperation I decided to apply my now more developed Ritual to my neck.

I placed my hands in the position shown in Fig.9.9 and began to focus the whole energy and emotion of my mind upon relieving the symptoms of pain in my neck, and upon increasing movement. I squeezed the muscles in my neck. I sensed the movement in the muscles beneath my fingertips and connected with it. I moved the focus of my mind beyond the muscles to the vertebrae beneath. I saw the vertebrae as plates stacked, white china plates, stacked neatly, fitting neatly one within the other. I affirmed how amazing the vertebrae in my neck were, how perfect and smooth and how effective at holding my neck.

I visualized the muscles in the neck as taut metal cords unwinding. I praised the neck muscles for all they had done in the past and for the good work they would do again. I applied therapeutic touch as demonstrated to maintain the connection between my neck and my mind. I did not expect sudden results and sudden results did not come but my injury was healed. My Ritual worked and I am still amazed. Within months of performing this exercise my neck was pain free, my old intractable injury and the pain that it caused me, history.

SNOW – BOARDING

Going down a mountain on a snow-board is like being strapped to a plank of wood and released on to a steep sheet of ice. Infact it is not like that. No need for a simile here. It is that. That is what snowboarding amounts to although the boards are not planks but thin and technically bonded sheets of poly carbon fibres fused together to ensure greater speed than any plank could deliver. The potential for injury is enormous. How I did not die or kill someone within my first years of snow-boarding will always remain for me a matter of fascination and marvel.

Throughout my snowboarding years I always felt on the edge of safety and then some years in to the sport on a piste I was unfamiliar with I lost control. I lost all ability to turn and careered towards an open ridge. I could do nothing to save myself but throw my body away from the precipice. My body complied but my board did not. Before my bindings released my ankle turned one way and my foot turned the other. I could not get my foot out of my boot. I was stretchered down the mountain and given a ride to the medical clinic on the 'blood wagon' but I did not even go inside. I put snow on the ankle. I sat watching the other boarders as they made their way down the slope and winced as I packed snow around my ankle bone.

I did not snow board again for two years but I snow board now. I did not go to the GP or the hospital X-ray clinic when I came home. I did not wait in line to hear the bones in my ankle had degenerated; that they showed signs of wear and tear. I did not want to be told the wrenching of my ankle in my fall had caused the onset of symptoms I would have experienced in any event, that I would now experience fifteen years sooner because of my injury intervening, disabling me, in the way I would have been disabled, at some point, when arthritis presented itself, as a result of the inevitable process of degeneration in our bones we all must face as we age.

I knew as I sat on the ski slope outside the medical clinic there was no point at all in going through the doors. I knew I had movement in my ankle, the very swollen joint could still be vaguely articulated and I knew with conviction the rest was down to me.

I began to focus my Ritual upon the ankle joint.

When I work with my ankle I work with my therapeutic massage applying the full force of the positive emotions held in my mind to the ankle joint. I visualise a perfect joint. It is helpful to create a powerful mental image that suggests strength and movement. I visualise a steel ratchet between my foot and my leg, oiled and freely moving.

I silently affirm how perfect and amazing my ankle joint is.

I believed when I commenced this exercise that by being totally mindful of the ankle joint it would respond to the Ritual and repair itself.

Pain free movement of the ankle joint was not immediate. Symptoms persisted for over six months. It was not until I was digging in my garden, applying the full weight of my foot and ankle to the task of pressing in the spade, I realised my ankle was no longer a problem. I realised it had not felt painful for some time and I realised with a real surge of delight, if my Ritual could settle my symptoms and have the effect upon my skeletal system it clearly had had, there was no reason why my Ritual could not keep me free from joint pain as I continued to age.

I felt suddenly resolute in my conviction that contemporary medicine could not deliver all the answers, quite simply because it had stopped looking for them. It became obvious, good health could not be delivered by GP's, consultants or specialists, who did not believe that after a certain age, good health was something that a man or woman could expect. A system that did not believe in vigorous longevity or dying in good shape simply did not see me as I wanted to be seen.

DIVING IN ACAPULCO

How I would love to be able to write that a swallow dive from a cliff in Guerrero Mexico just down the coast from Acapulco did not work out and that I damaged a ligament in my finger as I surfaced!

Well not quite!

I was in Acapulco and I was in the water but that's the nearest I get to the other set of facts. I tripped on a wave that broke just as I was walking from the beach in to the ocean. I fell on my outstretched hand and a ligament in my little finger snapped.

Now you will say, if I did not go in to the medical clinic in France when I fell while snowboarding there is absolutely no chance I would have gone anywhere near to a hospital waiting room with only a damaged finger.

Well perhaps that would have been true if I it were not for my passion for music. The little finger is essential in the positioning required for many guitar chords. I knew without my finger being repaired I could not play the guitar. I knew also that surgery would be required to attach the ligament back to the bone from which it had been wrenched.

It is my position throughout this book that we must live in the time in to which we are born and we must fully exploit every means our age delivers to sustain our lives and our health. I do not anywhere within this book propose that I would turn my back on the NHS if tomorrow a bomb exploded in my life ripping off a limb or I fell under a train.

I would not try to suggest I would be ok if someone made space for me to lie down and visualise and channel the best emotions I could draw from my mind to my injured body part. Of course not. I would gratefully accept help. I would accept whatever surgical procedure modern medicine could offer, whatever drugs, whatever routines but if I were physically capable, I would sustain the performance of my daily Ritual as a supplemental force to restore my being. Modern medicine and surgery would not cure me on its own, it would cure me as a result of all it provides and as a result of my will and determination to engage with the process of healing myself. The work I did on the damaged ligaments in my little finger, after surgical repair, convinces me I am right.

I went to hospital. I am blessed to live near to a hospital with a hand surgery unit which is recognised as excellent. I underwent an operation to repair my injured finger and when the ligament snapped a second time I underwent surgery again.

The problem with the cure delivered through the NHS was that the ligament was repaired. The finger had some movement within it. It could be straightened and the tip could be bent but it had lost most of the flexibility I needed to ever play the guitar, which was after all the only cure I desired.

I was discharged by my very excellent surgeon from ongoing hospital care, with regrets that fine manipulative tasks, and certainly guitar playing would no longer be possible in my life. I was so desperate to return to guitar playing I even attended the offered physiotherapy sessions, although I did not believe in them. My surgeon had threatened me with exclusion from her treatment programme if I did not attend and so I accepted my list of exercises and performed them dutifully to receive my physiotherapists assessment that I had 15% more movement in my injured finger than before physiotherapy commenced and that was the best I could expect. She was saddened I would not be able to play my guitar as I wished, but with her good wishes I was discharged.

I needed to play my guitar, it was a passion of my life, and that is where the Ritual came in.

Within around twelve to fourteen weeks of targeting the force of my Ritual upon my damaged finger I could curl my injured finger from tip to base, touching the base of my palm with my finger- tip.

I had questioned both physiotherapist and surgeon at length about the best means of restoring full movement within the finger. I had been told that due to the shortening of the ligament I would never have full movement within the finger and that I would ultimately adapt to the situation.

Well they were both wrong. I now not only curl my finger fully, holding the tip of my injured finger pressed against the strings of my guitar, I also perform complicated sequences of notes involving the damaged finger in deft and rapid sequences of movement as intricate as any fine manipulative task could be.

I am passionate about music. I play every morning. Music is for me energizing and uplifting. My mood changes when I play my music and the thought of not playing was quite frankly depressing. I was dejected but I simply was not prepared to believe the prognosis I had been given. At this stage in my life the Ritual had already displayed its transformative effect and I knew with all my heart if my Ritual were applied to my damaged hand full movement in my injured finger would return.

I believed 100% in the outcome the Ritual would deliver.

If I had been lying in intensive care I would not have believed the Ritual if applied would cause me to get up and walk but I would believe the Ritual would aid my recovery and trigger healing within me in ways tablets, surgical procedures, or therapy never could.

The effect of the Ritual is subtle and all pervading.

It is perhaps a last resort when mainstream medical intervention cannot achieve what it sets out to achieve. Perhaps the elements within the Ritual 'kick in' to bring a body back from the brink, to save a life, in circumstances where the only medical explanation is not a ritual but a miracle. Less dramatically the Ritual is a focused act of self care targeting the resources of the body and mind upon a particular problem with an intensity that simply is not achieved when a prescription is obtained or a pill taken.

THE RITUAL WORKS
BELIEVE IN IT AND IT WILL DELIVER ITS RESULTS.

PERSONALISING YOUR RITUAL FOR YOUR HEALTH

I have included a substantial number of exercises and photographs to depict the Ritual I perform. If you tried to perform each of the pictured exercises each and every day the Ritual would become overly demanding, dissatisfying and would inevitably within weeks be cast aside.

I restrict the time over which I practice the Ritual to a maximum of 45 minutes every day. On one day I may perform a face- lift and work out in the recumbent gym on another I may work through the exercises in Chapter 7.

After years of practising the Ritual I believe the important thing is to tailor the Ritual towards your own life, to how you are feeling. If life is sluggish and depressing, energise the nervous system, stimulate the brain. If you are lethargic or depressed, energise all the important organs and the lymph system. Alternate a full body Ritual with more specific work upon a part of the body that may be ailing you.

I used to suffer from recurring throat infections. I sing and singing places a lot of pressure on the throat and vocal chords. When it is winter and viruses are flying around my throat is vulnerable, as it is often over worked and so less resistant to infection. I make sure throughout winter at least on a couple of days a week I focus my Ritual upon my throat. It keeps me singing. No matter what science says. I get by without throat infections and laryngitis and to me that is all that counts.

I also have to admit I spent the best of two decades plagued by stomach ulcers and acid indigestion. I tell everyone that for longer than I remember my stomach was my bête noir. I spent prolonged periods ill, watching my diet, setting aside some foods in the hope of calming symptoms, refusing a glass of wine.

No more. I ensure that I perform the Ritual exercise I have created for my stomach, (as described earlier) each and every day. My stomach now is simply never a problem. I have a vague memory of the way in which I used to suffer and I am incredulous because today when it may be suggested I should avoid spicy food, as I am after all ageing and my juices are not flowing as they were, I ignore all advice and choose dishes full of chillies!

I have enjoyed holidays in Goa and Sri Lanka, where I not only survived but developed a real taste for the spice laden cuisine. Nor did I eat only in the safe anaesthetic environment of luxury hotels, I ate from street stalls and vendors on the beach!

I find devoting a few minutes of my daily Ritual to my stomach is the perfect prophylactic. My stomach Ritual if performed after a heavy meal or at the first sign of pains in the stomach is able to prevent any problem from developing. It also has a remarkably beneficial effect on both indigestion and bloating.

Take my advice and make the Ritual your own. You know the health problems that you have experienced and what may act to limit your actions in the future. Focus the Ritual upon the parts of your body that may in the past have let you down or render you vulnerable again at some point in the future.

We are all essentially the same and yet we all have our own individual health 'crosses' to bear. It is as if in the process of our creation minute flaws occur. The gift of the Ritual to your life is that it does not come pill shaped, with one set of blended chemicals within it obliged to be of benefit to every body on earth, the Ritual is your own therapeutic device, built by your mind to deal with any idiosyncracies of health your body may demonstrate.

PERSONALISING THE RITUAL FOR YOUR LIFE

MY SINGING VOICE

Just as we can tailor our Ritual to suit the ills that may weaken us so we can build our Ritual to support the individual gifts and talents we each display.

I am a singer. It is my hobby. Open MIC nights, making videos for You Tube, parties on holiday, playing my guitar on the beach, I enjoy them all. I practice every day.

As soon as I have finished my morning performance of the Ritual I go downstairs and pick up my guitar and play. It makes me feel good. A burst of loud singing, takes the blues away. It is absolutely impossible to be depressed when you are singing a happy song and enthusiastically engaged with projecting your voice.

Singing lesssons, piano lessons, guitar lessons, should be available on the NHS, (but that's another argument, not for developing now.)

The point is this, the Ritual has strengthened my voice. Ask any of my friends.

I would say fans, but they are generally one and the same!

Singing is tough on the throat and vocal chords, especially if you begin with Heartbreak Hotel! A whole lot of throat is involved!

Prior to practising the Ritual I could manage two or three songs, possibly four, but then my voice would begin to break up. I would be quite happy remaining in the limelight on the stage but I would just want to strum my guitar. Not recommended. Near riot ensues. No one understands if you get up to sing and display a kernel of talent that you cannot go on singing the whole night.

In the end my curtailed performances became too aggravating to those around me and my singing in public ceased.

Then I decided to apply my Ritual to my vocal chords.

I place my hands as shown in Fig 9.10

I place three fingers on one side of my throat, just under my jaw, breathe in, and exhale slowly.

The voice box is the top part of the human windpipe. We can all see and feel the front part of our larynx. It is what we

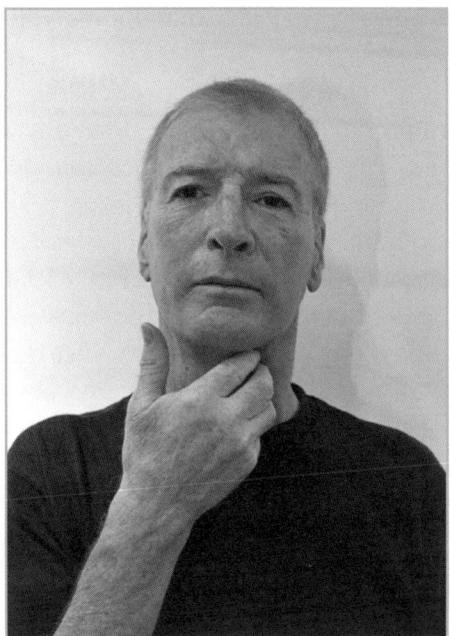

Fig 9.10

know as our Adam's apple on the front part of the neck, just below the chin. It is in this area that I place my three fingers.

Because my Ritual works through mind body connection, combined with mindful massage, exact anatomical positioning is not necessary. As I have set out in describing other exercises, applying therapeutic touch to the area proximate to the organ or structure of the body worked upon increases blood flow to that particular area with the consequent benefit of improving the functioning of the part of the body concerned.

By placing three fingers on one side of my throat just under my jaw I am near enough to the voice box to stimulate blood flow to this area. I AM ALSO VISUALLY CONNECTING and focusing my brain to carry positive energy and emotion to the top of my larynx.

I visualise how my perfectly functioning voice box would appear.

I tighten the muscles in my neck while focusing my visualisation upon my vocal chords. I see my vocal chords as frayed ropes smoothing themselves out. I visualise the fibres in the rope tightening and flattening. I silently affirm that there is no limit upon my voice or the notes I can sing. I hold my fingers in place as shown in Fig 9.10 and I feel the positive energy within the loving and compassionate emotion held in my mind being absorbed by my vocal chords.

I can literally sing all night, all my favourite songs, performed one after the other, even after practising for a full half-day. I have absolutely no doubt dedicating a small part of my daily Ritual to work on my vocal chords has strengthened my singing voice.

I stress it will work for you also. Feel no reticence, create a Ritual for your own life. Concentrate upon the Ritual exercises most likely to bring the most value to your own existence, to enhance the pursuits that you enjoy.

EXCITEMENT

As we arrive at the end of the chapters dedicated to presentation and explanation of the exercises within my Ritual let me say something about the approach I take to my daily Ritual performance.

In my mind as I perform my Ritual I simulate in my mind the excitement I might feel at achieving a great athletic triumph, a grand prix victory, olympic gold, winning the grand national. If you are of a literary bent imagine winning the Booker prize. Winning the lottery. The possibilities are endless, simulate excitement, transmit the excitement in your mind to the area of the body you are working on by mindfully tensing the tissues in the area beneath the skin. Localise the excitement to the part of your body you wish the Ritual to benefit.

As you tense and relax the tissues within you feel the release of all tension leaving. Imagine walking away with the prize, stepping down from the podium with a medal in your hand. It is that degree of satisfaction I want you to find. All the effort of the enterprise converted in to the joy of a victory and then relaxation.

What are we doing when we prepare ourselves in this way? What is the point of such wild visualising and elation?

IT IS ALL ABOUT ENDORPHINS.

Feel good. Feel excited. Feel alive. Stimulated. Believe in the Ritual you have created and the power within it. Anticipate the benefits your Ritual will deliver and feel the excitement generated by the prospect.

WHY?

Because it is like giving yourself an endorphin injection and endorphins are good for you.

—————————— CHAPTER TEN ——————————

WHY DOES THE RITUAL WORK?

So why does The Ritual work?
   Let's take a look at that.

THEORY ONE
SOMETHING DOES HAPPEN!

MY RITUAL HAS THE POWER WITHIN IT TO PROVOKE PHYSIOLOGICAL CHANGE IN THE BODY

In simple terms the placebo response, the response of the body to self –heal is not simply in our minds. The work of Fabrizio Benedetti and his colleagues at the University of Turin demonstrates that the placebo effect is not purely psychological but a phenomenon with biochemical physical consequences. What happens in the brain when a placebo pill is taken has been assessed using brain -imaging techniques. It is established science that the administration of a placebo results in objectively observable changes in a patient's brain, in terms of the activity of neurotransmitters, hormones and immune regulators. (1)

216

The experiments conducted by Benedetti et al at the University of Turin upon patients suffering with Parkinson's disease demonstrate a physical response to placebo medication and placebo procedures that can be evidenced on PET scans taken of the patient's brain.(2) Parkinson's patients given a placebo injection to alleviate symptoms of their condition, unaware they were receiving effectively a 'dummy' therapy, demonstrated raised levels of dopamine secretion in their brains, similar to that which could be expected from the administration of amphetamine.

In experiments conducted by Benedetti et al, in the mid 1990's, induced ischaemic pain in patients was relieved by administration of morphine. Morphine was then replaced by a placebo saline solution. Patients were not told of the change and the solution of simple salt and water continued to deliver an analgesic impact. The scientific team then added naloxone, an opiate antagonist, (a drug that reduces analgesic effect) to the saline. Results showed that the analgesic properties demonstrated by the saline were blocked.

Benedetti concluded that the analgesic properties of the saline resulted from the triggering of the same biochemical pathways in the brain as morphine. Naloxone blocked the action of endogenous opioids, nature's physical pain relievers, triggered by the act of administration of saline. (3)

Benedetti wrote of the findings in this experiment,

'What we placebo neuroscientists have learned is...that therapeutic rituals move a lot of molecules in the patient's brain, and these molecules are the very same as those activated by the drugs we give in routine clinical practice. In other words, rituals and drugs use the very same biochemical pathways to influence the patient's brain. (4)

Martina Amanzio, et al, through research conducted in 2001 demonstrated that *'at least part of the physiological basis for the placebo effect is opioid in nature.'* (5)

We can be conditioned to release endorphins, cortisol, adrenaline, in response to the action of swallowing a placebo pill. R Barker Bausell examined this aspect of our nature in *Snake Oil Science* published in 2007. (6) It is proposed that one reason people report pain relief from both acupuncture and sham acupuncture is that both are placebos that stimulate the opioid system, 'the body's natural pharmacy'.

Placebo induced endorphin release has been shown to affect a patient's heart rate and respiratory activity. The process of administration of a placebo produces a physical consequence in the heart and in the lungs. Nothing is given that can cause a bio chemical reaction in the body, it is the mind, and its reaction to the ritual of the offer and acceptance of a placebo pill that causes the body to react beneficially to absolutely nothing at all.

Further experiments conducted by Benedetti with Parkinson's patients demonstrated, *'objectively assessable, decreased activity, in neurons of the sub-thalmic nucleus in patients' brains when a placebo was administered.'* (7)

The changes in brain activity were, 'tightly correlated', with clinical improvement in the patients condition.

In patients suffering with depression variations have been witnessed in glucose metabolism similar to changes that could be expected when depressed patients are given biochemically active anti-depressants such as fluoxetine.

In 2006 and 2008 Ted Kaptchuk's team from Harvard carried out work to investigate the neural mechanisms of placebos in collaboration with the Martinos Centre for Biomedical Imaging at Massachusetts General Hospital. The results of two studies involving MRI imaging of the brains of placebo patients were published in the Journal of Neuroscience. The results showed placebo treatments affect the areas of the brain that determines how we react to pain. 'Nocebo' effects, that is the negative symptoms experienced by a patient resulting from the delivery of a placebo were shown, in the absence of any stimulus from any active drug, to affect the part of the brain called the hippocampus, the area of the brain associated with memory and anxiety. (8)

The knowledge that the body has the power to physiologically react to inert placebo substances is not sudden new positioning within the world of placebo science. In 1949 placebo researchers were convinced that something tangible happened to the body when a placebo was given. One of the first proponents to accept that the impact of placebo medication was not simply psychological was Stewart Wolf, in 1949 he wrote;

'the mechanisms of the body are capable of reacting not only to direct physical and chemical stimulation but also to symbolic stimuli, words and events, which have somehow acquired a special meaning for the patient.' (9)

The potential of a placebo to impact upon the body of the patient in physiological terms, inducing biological change as a consequence of a patient swallowing thin air or submitting to surgery as effective as a rub with a towel, is evident from the results of a placebo experiment constructed to persuade patients to believe they had been infected with hazardous bacilli.(10)

The patients in this experiment were informed that treatment was necessary to stem the expected spread of infection that afflicted them and treatment was given. The medication given was a placebo as the patients were not in fact ill and had not been infected. Despite this some of the trial subjects developed infection like symptoms that were not treatable with the placebo medication. They *'presented as sick and appeared genuinely unwell.'* Scientists concluded that the minds of those made ill interpreted the fictional bacilli as hazardous and instructed the body to respond to them as if they were real.

So, what has any of this got to do with my Ritual?

Quite simply this, I believe my Ritual acts as effectively as any placebo to promote a physical response within the systems, cells, and structures of my body that is beneficial to my health.

My belief in a positive outcome from performance of my Ritual is reinforced by my daily act of performance. I make my Ritual important, I set aside time. Following a prescribed set of actions, in a set pattern, in an established way, converts my therapeutic act, in to a ritual my brain responds to.

The work of the placebo scientists persuades me that my Ritual is promoting beneficial physiological change within the structures of my body without the need for any pharmacologically active or rapaciously - marketed but otherwise useless cosmetic substance being taken or applied.

My body I am persuaded is responding to my strongly held conviction that my Ritual promotes good health. The biological consequences of my Ritual are not within my imagination; they are substance and reality stemming from the action I take every morning to communicate with, energise and empower the body that I have.

THEORY TWO.

NEUROPLASTICITY.

It came as a revelation to me that my brain is not an unchanging organ. It is not physiologically static but an organ that alters shape and structure with the experiences and activities of life. Did any one else realise this to be the case or did you like me consider the brain to be an unchanging mass? If you did we are both entirely wrong. Science has demonstrated our every experience, injury, and activity, changes the shape and structure of our brain throughout every day of our lifetime.

Adopt a different activity, for example, oil painting, or clay modelling and the area of the brain required for the newly sought activity will develop.

This concept of the reactive changing brain is known as neuroplasticity. The practice of meditation has been shown to change the density of both grey matter and white matter in the brain, to increase cortical thickness and impact beneficially upon the hippocampus.(11)

Flexing even one finger repeatedly for a considerable period of time will change the structure of the part of the brain involved in movement of our fingers. More astoundingly, even *imagining* movement of one finger of the hand, repeated over a prolonged period of time, will change the structures within the brain involved with finger movement.

Thought alone can impact on the form, structure and activity of the brain. Thought triggers a movement of blood and oxygen, the chemistry of the brain changes, which initiates physical change in the brain. Physical change results from chemical change and an alteration of the brain's chemistry can be triggered by altered thought. (12)

The hippocampus, the part of the brain holding spatial representation information is more developed in London taxi drivers compared to London bus drivers driving similar routes. (13)

Taxi drivers exercise the hippocampus to find diversions and speedier routes whereas bus drivers following a programmed route do not.

In the Moken, a sea faring people surviving from fishing the seas off Thailand, the pupil in their eyes was found to be 22% restricted leading to an acuity of vision in a land of piercing light and water not seen in those who do not fish or scan the seas for a catch.(14)

The Moken study demonstrates the ability of the body to adapt to survive, the ability of the brain to re-size, re-shape and alter activity, to respond to individual needs and the information that is fed in to it.

My mantra, expressed without reservation, is that I AM AWESOME, that I have the power within me never to be ill. I hold this fact in my mind. I believe it one hundred percent. I really do believe I can engineer my future life longevity and happiness by changing the thoughts that I have and by stimulating the most effective communication possible between my mind and my physical being.

Understanding something about the nature of neuroplasticity I am convinced that the Ritual is promoting change at a cellular level and that the change my Ritual delivers is beneficial. Incorporation of my Ritual in to my day has changed the information my mind has to deal with and it is I believe this change from negative to overwhelmingly positive programming that is delivering results.

Scientific studies confirm the brain to be remarkably adaptive and 'plastic'. Studies of the brains of stroke victims have demonstrated the ability of the brain to re-organise itself. (15) To move body function from the stroke affected regions of the brain to the direction of undamaged areas.

The number of neurons in our brain is ever changing. Exercise and cognitive stimulation changes the number of new cells our brain creates. Neuroplasticity demonstrates our ability to shape our brains, and ' with our ability to shape our brains, comes the ability to shape our destiny',(16)

Brain training courses are available on the Internet. I have never tried them but I do not doubt they have the capacity to work to increase cognitive ability by requiring the brain to 'exercise'. Prisoners of war detained in camps in the Second World War demonstrated very significant developments in cognitive capacity. Upon release many were found to have unusual gifts mathematically. The prisoners could for example deal with long equations or multiply correctly a 12 digit number by any other random 12 digit number and arrive at the correct answer. The theory goes that all the prisoners could do when incarcerated was think and endeavour to retain their sanity by the only mental stimulation available to them, mental mathematics.

A well reported and inspiring study in to the plasticity of the brain is the Harvard Piano Study. (17) Trial participants were divided in to two groups. One group of would be pianists was told to play a group of notes on the piano as fluidly as they could. They were asked to practice the notes and play the piece of music given to them repetitively for 2 hours a day over a period of 5 days. After 5 days brain scans were taken of this group of participants. The scans revealed the area of the motor cortex involved in finger movement had massively increased in size.

The second group of trial participants did not play the piano but they imagined playing it. While holding their hands together they imagined playing the same group of notes as those played by participants in group one, over the same time, 2 hours a day, over five days. Remarkably the area of the motor cortex involved in finger movement also dramatically increased in size, in this non-playing group, to the same extent as those actually moving their fingers and really playing the piece on the piano. In other words *thought alone* had the same impact upon the structure of the brain as physical action, demonstrating that thought held has the power to change the physical structures within our brains.

Those involved in sports science immediately leapt upon the piano trial results as demonstration that visualising a perfect golf swing or a forward football pass could dramatically improve performance in sport, leading to a mastery of skills with less physical practice.

I leap upon the Harvard piano study results to say this; if the area of the brain responsible for organisation of our lymph system, endocrine and immune system can be developed in a similar way through visualisation of each system performing in optimal fashion, and affirmation of the good health, high energy levels, and resistant immunity, we anticipate, would that not have an impact on the quality and longevity of our lives?

For me there is no doubt that the results of such visualisation would be beneficial.

Neuroplasticity is exciting because it allows us to take control. When we understand that we are capable of changing our brains, by changing our activities and the thoughts that we hold, we understand we are not helpless participants within our own lifetime but instead orchestrators of the life that we have, the health we hold on to, the passion we retain for living and new pursuits.

The concept of neuroplasticity convinces me, that what is, in effect, my act of brainwashing myself through affirmation, positivity and repeatedly stated beliefs has caused changes within my brain at a bio chemical and structural level.

This change in body chemistry engendered by no more than the thoughts which I hold, has I believe beneficially altered my brain and body chemistry improving the health I experience, the outlook I have, the energy within me and the rate at which I am ageing.

THEORY THREE

THE RITUAL CHANGES THE ENERGETIC ENVIRONMENT OF THE CELLS WITHIN MY BODY DELIVERING ASTOUNDING BENEFITS FOR MY HEALTH

To have any idea what sub-heading three means it is necessary to be acquainted with the work of Dr Bruce Lipton, and his outstanding work, *The Biology of Belief.* (18)

Dr Bruce Lipton is a cellular biologist and research scientist. His work *The Biology of Belief* considers the manner our cellular health, the foundation if you like of our health, is dictated by the environment we create for our cells through our activities thoughts and beliefs. Dr Lipton proposes that the behaviour and activity of a cell is influenced by more than genes and DNA. It is Dr Lipton's argument that each of us, the individual possessor of the cells within our body, has a role to play in the creation of cell environment.

If Dr Lipton's proposition is correct we have a suddenly announced and indeed somewhat extraordinary degree of control over the health that we possess.

We are freed from the notion our health is dictated by the genes that we inherit. Within *The Biology of Belief,* Dr Lipton unites the principles of quantum physics with those of cellular biology to present a science which burdens us with responsibility for creating the shape that we are in and the future we grant to ourselves.

We can take control, that is the clear message Dr Bruce Lipton's work provides. Dr Lipton instructs us that cellular health, cellular activity and cellular responses are affected by a cellular environment *we create* as we live our life. Even more helpfully he tells us that cellular environment is influenced and can be changed by a change in our activities, our actions, our beliefs and our thoughts.

The suggestion that our genes and our DNA do not control our biology is liberating. The concept that we have a degree of control, that our essential structure, our DNA, is not code that cannot be overwritten but genetic code that can be changed by our actions and the thoughts we entertain, is both revelatory and challenging. It is a thesis entirely supportive of my contention that a ritual, and for the purposes of this book, my Ritual, has the power within it to change the being that I am, by changing the thoughts and information I feed in to my brain.

Bruce Lipton writes:

A cell's life is controlled, by the physical and energetic environment of the cell ; with only a small contribution by the cells genes. Genes are simply molecular blueprints used in the construction of cells tissues and organs. The environment serves as a contractor who reads and engages those genetic blueprints and is ultimately responsible for the character of a cell's life.

Our human environment is that internal to our being, our gender, hormones, and metabolism. Our predetermined coded substrate, but environment is more than that. It is also the environment we impose upon our cells through the diet we eat, the level of exercise we take, the level of stress we subject our bodies to, the level of toxins we allow in to our lives and the number of medicines we take. Such factors impact upon the physical environment constructed for our cells. Professor Lipton advises us that our thoughts and beliefs impact upon the energetic environment of a cell.

Clearly we cannot affect our predetermined sex, the balance of our hormones, but we can directly affect all external matters, which impact upon cell environment. We can alter our diet, the medicines we take, the toxins to which we are exposed. We are in control of our thoughts and beliefs. We can think differently and we can act differently at any chosen time.

We can for example decide to engage in a contemplative Ritual every morning of our life. Slow down our heartbeat, let in a sense of calm. Change our mind set from bleak to optimistic by flooding in positive thoughts. Current biological science is handing us control. If we change our environment we can change our gene response. If we change our gene response we change our ability to maintain, repair and sustain the being we are.

Eminent scientist and physician Dean Ornish (*Ornish et al 2008*) (19) has through his research demonstrated that just by changing the diet and lifestyle of prostate cancer patients over a period of 90 days, prostate cancer patients switched the activity of over 500 genes. Many of their gene changes inhibited biological processes critical in the formation of their tumours.

After reading of the work of Dean Ornish and *The Biology of Belief* I am persuaded that my morning Ritual has the potential to impact upon the energetic environment I create for the cells within every organ, structure and system of my body.

I believe the Ritual combined with the habits and routines that amount to the *other secrets* of my life, (set out in Chapter 14), promote beneficial changes in my cellular environment with demonstrable consequences for my life.

THEORY FOUR
OUR BODY AND NOT JUST OUR MIND IS WISE.

Candace Pert was a brilliant neuroscientist. She sadly died in the autumn of 2013 but she leaves the legacy of her very substantial body of scientific work to all of mankind. In particular her wonderful and compelling treatise presented in *Molecules of Emotion- Why You Feel The Way That You Feel.* (20)

Candace Pert was, for many years, Research Professor in the Department of Physiology and Biophysics at Georgetown University Medical Centre in Washington DC. She is known as the scientist who identified the opiate receptor in the brain. Her work *Molecules of Emotion* is one of the leading scientific works to explain the role of emotions in health and to connect the thoughts that we hold and the feelings we possess with the state of our health and well - being.

Candace Pert explored how emotion could transform the body, either by creating disease, or by healing it, by maintaining health or undermining it. Candace Pert recounts studying the process of bio- feedback. Quoting, Elmer Green, a physician in the Mayo Clinic in the United States, a scientist studying systems of bio-feedback, she writes (21);

'Every change in the physiological state is accompanied by an appropriate change in the mental, emotional state, conscious or unconscious, and conversely, every change in the mental emotional state, conscious, or unconscious, is accompanied by an appropriate change in the physiological state'.

Candace Pert dedicated much of her scientific research to understanding systems of information within the body and the means by which messages are exchanged between cells and different biological systems. Her work disabuses us of the notion that mind body communication is a one way system of messaging which emanates from the brain sending messages by means of electrical impulses across synapses to other body parts.

Candace Pert describes a system of information exchange between organs, systems and structures within the body, which relies upon intelligent bio chemical messengers to transfer and carry information. This information exchange, she tells us, triggers activity within cells, guiding our life and our health.

Candace Pert was effectively describing a second chemically based 'nervous system'. A system of communication between substances within the body and cells allowing for bio-chemical messages to be transferred not only between mind and body but between body and mind. In her work she describes peptides travelling in extra- cellular space and in blood and spinal fluid, acting as bio- chemical messengers, intelligently communicating information and stimulating complex and fundamental changes within cells themselves. This secondary system of information allows not just the mind but cells to communicate across every important system the body has, including the endocrine, gastrointestinal, neurological, and immune system.

Candace Pert provides us with the concept of the 'mobile brain'. Of a brain not situated within the head but within every organ structure and system of the body across which information is exchanged. She describes the body-mind, making us think differently about the manner in which our body and mind communicate.

Candace Pert believed the complex molecular biochemical structures existing on the surface of cells formed the *'physiological substrate of emotion, underpinning what we experience as thoughts, drives, sensations, feelings'*.

Candace Pert even went as far to suggest that the bio-chemicals she described could form the physical substrate of spirit or soul.

I find the writing of Candace Pert overwhelmingly positive as to the potential we all have to command our body, directing it towards health.

Her theories result from years of research carried out in the confines of a scientific laboratory but they transport her far beyond the walls of any science laboratory to an elevated plane, that exists somewhere beyond pure science. Through her lifetime of research Candace Pert arrived at the interface of science, philosophy, belief and spirituality. Candace Pert proposed that full consciousness was not only mental consciousness but also emotional consciousness. To be fully conscious was to be aware of the body to such an extent that one could almost listen in to bodily systems.

As she put it:

'the more conscious we are, the more we can 'listen in' to the conversation going on at autonomic or subconscious levels of the bodymind, where basic functions, such as breathing, digestion, immunity, pain control and blood flow are carried out. Only then can we enter in to that conversation, using our awareness to enhance the effectiveness of the autonomic system, where health and disease are being determined minute by minute'. (22)

I believe Candace Pert was right. I believe bio -chemical messages can be re-written and changed by firstly communing with yourself and then by recognition, acceptance and release of damaging and limiting emotions stored at a level of memory within cells.

The Ritual is, I suggest, a powerfully contemplative process that allows us to enhance communication between our mind and our body. The communion my Ritual proposes is between the body and a mind of greater dimensions than has ever been described to me by anyone other than Candace Pert. It is a mind not positioned within the head but within every cell, in every organ, every bone, and every fluid the body has.

The fact of a 'bodymind' made immediate sense to me of the practice, I had begun instinctively, that of praising and congratulating the different parts of myself. 'Chatting' as it were, to every organ within me. To, my liver, heart, spleen, praising and encouraging the work that was being done, before moving on to celebrate, my pancreas, my lymph nodes, my lungs and every other structure, and substance I come across as my Ritual completes its bodily rounds .

I now have absolutely no doubt my Ritual enhances the degree of successful intervention I achieve in the ongoing conversation of my bodily self.

Candace Pert tells us of a psychic invocation she was taught by a friend (23) and urged to use at moments when she was down or in need of protection. Candace Pert tells us reciting the words of the invocation made her feel protected and delivered a sort of strength. Initially Candace Pert put this down to the psychological buffering from injury performing the invocation provided until she realised the power of what was effectively a charm came not from psychology but from the consequences of reciting the words. Candace Pert describes the invocation working by means of an, *'extra corporeal peptide reaching'*. Which she explains, is an experience of emotional resonance, that happens when receptors are vibrating together in seemingly separate systems.

I find this explanation moving and compelling because to me it comes the closest in scientific terms to describing what my Ritual is doing.

My Ritual is applied outside the body but it has a resonance within, which is powerful and life changing. My Ritual may be as easy to discredit as your average charm but this does not diminish its effect, or the power that it has.

THEORY FIVE.

MY RITUAL WORKS BECAUSE I BELIEVE IT WILL WORK

I could not omit from Chapter 10, this chapter of synthesis of ideas explored in an effort to understand the mechanics and effectiveness of my Ritual, the concept of belief.

Belief, defined by Thomas Aquinas, as, *'the intellectual assent to truths, accepted on authority, either human or divine,'* delivers solutions.

Indeed to believe, to have faith in some deity or other has been shown to have real health benefits and to be as effective as belief in a doctor or a pill.

Spirituality has been considered an overlooked predictor of placebo effects.

'*Assessment of patients' spirituality...making use of resources to accommodate patients' spiritual needs....may increase the likelihood of eliciting self healing processes'.*

'*Ongoing studies suggest that spiritual experiences and practices involve a variety of neural systems that may facilitate neural 'top-down' effects that are comparable if not identical to those engaged in the placebo response'.* (24)

Paolo Lissoni of the San Gerardo Hospital in Milan conducted a study of patients with advanced lung cancer to determine if the impact of administered chemotherapy could be enhanced by the use of the hormone melatonin and to consider comparative healing rates between patients with a real developed spiritual faith and those without faith. (25)

The percentage of objective tumour regression obtained in patients with a high degree of spiritual faith was significantly higher than that found in other patients concomitantly treated with chemo and hormone therapy.

What then divides the devout, kneeling upon their knees in prayer and the patient in the waiting room full of the firmly held belief that the physician who is to attend upon him will heal?

I contend very little.

Both believe; belief in a divine outcome recognised and praised as spiritual faith. Belief in a GP or consultant considered acceptable credence in someone vested with medical authority, enabled by training and expertise to act as a conduit to health.

It is demonstrably the case that both drugs and surgery work better if patients believe in the pill given or the method invoked for healing. Placebo experiments involving sugar pills and cunningly constructed fake surgical procedures have demonstrated this time and time again.

Belief is I believe the agent that makes the difference, quietening a soul, delivering salvation, or halting the onslaught of disease.

Patients with severe debilitating knee pain who succumbed to the phoney arthroscopy procedure performed in an operating theatre in 2002 by Dr Bruce Moseley believed absolutely the procedure Dr Moseley offered to them would reduce knee pain or they would not have submitted to the routine.

The outcome for those deceived, who had surrendered themselves to surgery, to receive in the end, only knife pricks and puffs of fresh air, was the same as for those operated upon, in terms of pain free movement and reduction of disability.

An assessment of Dr Moseley's patients was carried out at multiple points over a 24 month period following the completion of the trial and overall the benefits in terms of pain relief and joint function for those receiving arthroscopy of the knee were no better than that achieved in the placebo group. (26)

The outcome for the NHS is clear. If belief can achieve the same as one of the most used orthopaedic procedures in modern medicine, billions of pounds are probably best spent elsewhere. Indeed I would suggest the funds for arthroscopic surgery are best re- routed, immediately, within any health system, to placebo research.

Moreover to harness the power of a patient's belief, should modern medicine not change?

Should there not be some revision of ethical guidelines for the dispensing of medicine or the offer of a surgical procedure, to allow the inculcation of belief, when demonstrably belief heals?

In 2009, even more dramatically than the experience of those undergoing placebo arthroscopic surgery two concurrently published studies showed that vertebroplasty (a technique in which a polymer cement is injected in to the spine) was no more effective than a placebo in relieving symptoms of pain caused by spinal compression. (27)

In the vertebroplasty experiments 130 patients were treated. In the placebo control group all aspects of vertebroplasty surgery to inject cement in to the spine were simulated. The patient was injected with a local anaesthetic. The button on the pump used to introduce cement in to the spinal canal was pressed.

One half of the patients treated received an injection of polymer. In the other half of the patient group nothing was injected although the button on the polymer pump could be seen by the patient treated to be depressed.

Patients had no idea which group of patients they had been assigned to. The one thing they had in common was their belief that a vertebroplasty was being carried out and they as patient were engaged in the performance.

Remarkably those receiving an injection of cement fared no better in terms of pain relief or increased mobility than those receiving thin air. In one case a woman who had undergone an earlier vertebroplasty and received no benefit from it, was very significantly improved by the repeated procedure, recovering a large degree of mobility and returning to her passion, golf, even though she was in the group of patients assigned to receive nothing at all. Her life was transformed not by cement but by belief.

On the 17th February 2014, *Horizon*, the long running BBC science series broadcast the results of placebo trials conducted by Dr Chris Beedie from the University of Aberystwyth.

Dr Chris Beedie is reported to have stated. (28)

'Our research findings suggest that performance levels similar to those resulting from drugs can be achieved through a placebo', 'In short the mind is at play as much as the body when an athlete uses drugs'.

Dr Beedie and his team examined what happened to athletes when they were told they had taken a performance -

enhancing drug containing large amounts of caffeine, when in fact the tablet given was a placebo. Athletes improved their performance, some obtaining personal bests in time trials even though nothing was in their system that could have had an effect upon their speed or the results obtained.

The brain of the high performing athletes clearly believed the athlete would deliver an enhanced performance as a result of taking a powerful experimental drug and, what do you know? The record breaking performance was delivered.

It is a matter of some fascination to me that the same athletes told they had been given a drug that would hamper their performance, slowing them down, acted as expected, delivering worse results, as the 'nocebo' effect of the harmless pill taken came in to play. The athletes delivered a poor performance to accord with their firmly held belief that the tablet they had been given would slow them down, although there was no chemical within the tablet that could deliver a bio chemical effect of any relevance to the performance they gave.

I believe as I begin my Ritual my body will be more energised throughout the remainder of my day than if my Ritual was not performed. I believe every organ system and structure in my body will remain disease free and function at its most effective because of the attention I pay to the body part I engage with as my Ritual is performed. I don't just pay lip service to the fact my Ritual is delivering my health. I believe it 100% with an unshakeable conviction that has developed within me over the years my Ritual has been performed.

My belief is now so firmly held I am boringly evangelical about the power my Ritual has. It is why this book is written. My health, my enhanced level of energy and my ability to perform as I do at my age are as much testament to my belief as they are to any other aspect of my invented routine.

THEORY SIX

THE RITUAL WORKS BECAUSE IT IS A RITUAL AND RITUALS ARE EFFECTIVE IN DELIVERING HEALTH BENEFITS

Go back to theory one at the beginning of this chapter. Remember that Fabrizio Benedetti told us:

' *Therapeutic Rituals move a lot of molecules in the patient's brain'*

I think it is important to examine the power of ritual. The organising of therapy in to component parts, each of which must be followed and acted out, if the ritual in question is to be effective.

The Navajo created entire dramas populated with characters and song to enact the healing rituals of their nation. The act of healing was a theatrical presentation involving the patient and the healer and a host of other characters. The whole of the culture, ancestry and mysticism of a people were involved in casting out illness. How could a Navajo not be healed when the might of a nation was brought down to treat or expel an individual malaise.

Ted Kaptchuk analyses therapeutic rituals, their respective dimensions, power and effects, in a comparative study of the rituals within Navajo healing ceremonies, chinese acupuncture and western bio medical treatment. (29)

Ted Kaptchuk presents his opinion that placebo effects, often described as, 'non specific', in modern medicine are in fact, the ' specific' effects of healing rituals.

It was important to me to create a Ritual that I could peform every morning. This gave form and structure to my belief that communing with myself, laying my hands upon my body in an orchestrated sequence of movement, while engaging my brain to the task of restoration and repair was a means of transferring energy between my brain and my body, of stimulating a response, of 'waking up' dormant cells and rejuvenating processes that were slowing down.

In creating my Ritual it felt appropriate to set aside time, to lie down in a quiet space, to relax my brain and focus the whole of my attention upon my healing task, before beginning the pattern of movements performed with my hands which have become as natural to me as the steps of a dance.

Each part of the process of my Ritual has meaning for me, the consequence being, a part, an action, cannot be omitted from my daily act. My Ritual has developed the innate power rituals contain. To change one part of the process, to attempt to perform my Ritual piecemeal, in several parts, or casually or not at all would affect my energy, exuberance, outlook, and the health that I possess.

Writing of the neurological consequences rituals have for the body, Ted Kaptchuk states:

'Rituals have neurobiological correlates. This suggests that patient improvement is not only report bias or desire to please the healer but represents changes in neurobiology. Specific areas of the brain are activated and specific neurotransmitters and immune markers may be released' (30)

He concludes,

'At a minimum, healing rituals provide an opportunity to reshape and recalibrate selective attention. In a more expanded model, rituals trigger specific neurobiological pathways that specifically modulate bodily sensations, symptoms and emotions. It seems that if the mind can be persuaded, the body can sometimes act accordingly'. (31)

I believe the very act of shaping my daily programme in to a therapeutic Ritual has magnified the effectiveness of the therapy I have developed. Every aspect of my daily routine is rich with meaning for me and significant to different aspects of my health. My repetition of positive empowering affirmations combined with visual imagery and meditative massage is as important in my life as energy meridians to the Chinese or chant pathways to the Navajo.

The casually created practice begun many years ago with cursory stomach massage has developed in to a tightly constructed and developed healing practice.

In his paper, *Examining a Powerful Healing Effect through a Cultural Lens, and finding Meaning,* Moerman writes:

'If placebos do not do anything, then it seems possible that what we call, 'placebo effects', might occur without placebos' (32)

I am with him, I believe my Ritual does what a placebo pill does, effectively as a consequence of the mysterious potential of rituals.

CHAPTER ELEVEN

POSITIVITY

THE BENEFITS OF A POSITIVE MINDSET

If by this stage, after reading all that is written to this point, you find merit in the idea of the Ritual, you may even have begun to create a daily Ritual for yourself. I have said throughout that my Ritual as organised by me is not prescriptive. I have provided the elements of my own Ritual performance and it is now for every person who wishes to, to tailor the Ritual for themselves.

When I began the Ritual I could not know how my health would be five years down the line. I could not know that my energy levels instead of depleting would increase, that instead of having one life goal of narrow purpose I would have several, that in the intervening period I would be illness, disease and virus free. I nevertheless engaged with the Ritual positively. I foresaw great things, bathing myself in positivity as I created the different steps my Ritual now has.

It is important that I stress this because together in this book we are unravelling a mystery, the mystery of self healing; of maintenance and repair of the body we possess. Whatever the secret combination of elements that leads to the one result, the joyousness of enduring good health, vigour, energy, and purpose, regardless of chronological age, positivity undoubtedly has a role to play.

To be positive, is not to be ridiculous, to coast about, in an irritating state, slapping others on the back, oblivious to the problems of the world in which we all live.

Positivity is the opposite. It is a grounded and powerful state that harnesses energy. Positivity is centred in reality, it is a way of seeing the facts infront of a person and adjusting the mental response the brain delivers to one of constructive engagement. We all are older than we were ten or twenty years ago.

So what?

Why is it that *en masse* we consider ageing to be a negative?

Let us carry out an experiment in to the power of the positive.

Let us use positivity to reconstruct our opinion of age?

Ageing in the early part of our lives is about empowerment; why in later decades is that outlook not sustained?

In my opinion it is down to a combination of three principal events.

The impoverishment of our lives financially as we cease to earn. Encroaching disability as our body begins to let us down. The insidious sidelining that takes place as the society around us decides we no longer have a useful contribution to make.

No wonder we do not look at ageing in positive terms. No wonder we see our purposive lives as ceased and our role reduced to spiralling downwards towards our end.

The very thoughts we construct about ageing change the future that we get. The negative opinions and beliefs we harbour about life as we age can deliver only one thing; the bleak reality that has been forseen, of dependence, deprivation and care.

The important thing to realise is that we can change what we receive. And the quickest way to change our reality is to change our thinking. It is within our gift to change our mindset, and in changing our mindset to change the future that is delivered.

We can even change the view society takes of those who are aged. The present opinion society has of the elderly is based upon past experience. The envisaged future predicted for those post retirement can only be cast and made real if every elderly person in society engages with the presently presented stereotypes. If there is a refusal to engage and an insistence upon reversing all set opinions, present stereotypes will dissolve in to myth.

In my opinion by the time we come to retire too many of us have forgotten who we actually are. Too many of us have lost our identity within our work. We are not the architect who designed all the houses on Woolmer Row, we are George or Iris. We are not the lorry driver who used to drive from the edge of Birmingham to Vigo in ten and a half hours, we are Eddy or Louise. We are not our work. We are the collection of cells that turned up for the job but we are and always will be, us, the entity quite separate to any employment we have had.

The most crucial time to realise this is when retirement begins.

Not many of us have adequate pensions to replace the income we have grown used to during our working life. As the decades unfold, more and more of us will have substantially less money upon which to live. It is not likely in our retirement the majority of us will be able to buy the same cars, or enjoy the same holidays we became used to when we worked. Too many of us living in the later part of the 20th century have used our earnings to support our every day lives. The good news being, we are not going to be on our own in our pension crisis!

Its all about the way that the facts delivered are considered.

Who can say what society will look like in ten or twenty years as the elderly begin to tip the boat and in their vast surviving numbers hold sway in a democracy that must listen to what the voters want. It is not necessarily going to be bleak for any of us living at present, it could indeed for many of us, be the first time, in political terms, we have held real power.

Family groupings may change as they are changing now. Today children leave home after the age of 30 if they leave at all. Economics dictates that. Economics may also dictate that parents return, selling what is possessed to buy a bigger space with their children or pooling pension and other state benefits in a home that is shared. Pensioners who have been friends for a lifetime may decide to move in together or buy a new house. The housing market may have to take a new shape. The saying, 'you cannot choose your family, but you can choose your friends', may lead to happier co-habitations and Christmases than ever previously seen!

What I am saying is this. There are a myriad of ways of looking at the likely impoverishment of age and a myriad of ways in which the brain can construct solutions if positive energy is engaged to look at what, many may consider a depressing situation, in a different way.

Let's look at disability. Today those in their sixties are considered to still be young, fit, able, productive, not necessarily retired. Indeed those in their seventies are not considered to be old. They are on the margins of old age; still recognised as not in need of support, perhaps still in work, living independently, still travelling, enjoying holidays and the world. Seventy is the beginning of age but it is certainly not old. What about 80, how is 80 regarded?

Those in their 80's, are admittedly, likely to be considered as aged. Increasing in fragility. In need of support. Unlikely to be working but not unlikely to be living in their own home. As many eighty year olds are able to live independently as in sheltered accommodation or in care. A percentage of those over eighty are still driving and mobile. A percentage indeed are still occupied with work, particularly the self employed with business interests from which they are unwilling to disengage.

The map of age has changed dramatically in as little as twenty years.

In the next ten or twenty years it will change again as the ruler slides and those in their late seventies are in good shape, those in their eighties need less support, the bar raised until the age of the aged is that of those near or approaching ninety.

Our present society does not make sense. You must realise that. It is now quite ridiculous to have those in public office allowed to receive a pension at the age of 55. At 55 we are not pensionable we are in the midst of our lives.

The recent panic driven changes to the minimum retirement age for men and women demonstrate the sudden recognition that we are fitter longer and retired much longer than was ever forseen.

Now that you have purchased the Ritual and are overhauling your approach to your health and to the rest of your life it is important to engage positively with the age that you have and to recognise if you are in your sixties or indeed early seventies, you are not old. We are evolved to a state in which those in their sixties or seventies, are on balance, all things being equal, and allowing for the life changes that will be made subsequent to buying this book, going to live longer and in better health, with more retained ability than future generations have ever been able to display.

So let's look at the correlate between age and disability in a different way?

That is let us disabuse ourselves of notion number two, that for those retiring or about to retire a diminished future of increasing disability is all that awaits.

I stress the way in which society regards the aged is within the gift of the aged. Stereotypical opinions and attitudes towards the elderly are likely to change if those in their sixties seventies and eighties instead of falling in to dependency maintain their energy and drive for life. If those nearing or at retirement age are full of energy, ill less, active more, with plans and projects and talents that remain of use and benefit to all around them, how are the aged going to be regarded, but with awe?

If you have bought this book as you are wondering what shape your retirement will take; what purpose your life can have now that you have ceased an occupation that you have so long considered part and parcel of what you are, take heart. The good news is, we are all still here.

Modern health care, sanitation, a prolonged period of peace between nations and raised standards of accommodation, better standards of safety, better regulation of energy and the environment, all mean we have reached old age in good shape. It is now up to all who are retired or about to retire to take the next decades in to their hands and build a long, stable and joy filled future upon the scaffolding provided.

It is time to recognise the power of the positive and to reverse in the brain every fact that is likely to place ageing in a negative light. Think of age as a time to be wise. To see life differently, to engage with living in a different way. Think of the richness in experience, the power it equips any person with. Later life need not be a poorer experience, considered positively, and seen for what they really are, the last decades of life can be the best, the ones worth waiting for.

How are you feeling after this positive pep talk?

Are you willing to engage positively with your life?

What about your energy levels? Are they raised, are you willing to stand up, cast off all negativity and head out to an old age full of challenge and adventure?

I should hope so.

At the very least I would hope you are feeling more optimistic about what later life may present.

Your mood, outlook and level of happiness should have changed, not just for one reader, but for all readers. How can I know this. How can I confront you with how your emotions are as you reach the bottom of this page.

Because human beings are all the same. They have built in to them fundamentally similar response mechanisms. The human brain lights up and fires differently when fuelled by positivity.

Positivity is good for you!

What is more positivity is seen as so relevant in delivering health benefits it is now considered a science in itself. Courses on positive psychology abound. Academic papers provide insight in to how positivity works.

A landmark paper written by B.L Fredrickson (1) describes the increasing resourcefulness developed by those who exude and display positivity. Fredrickson proposes that positive emotions have significant consequence for human welfare and health. Not just as indicators or marks of health and well –being but as *producers* of health.

Fredrickson writes:

Put differently, to the extent that the broaden and build effects of positive emotions accumulate and compound over time, positive emotions carry the capacity to transform individuals for the better, making them healthier and more socially integrated, knowledgeable, effective and resilient. In short, the theory suggests that positive emotions fuel human flourishing'.

In a separate paper written by Barbara Fredrickson, Michelle Tugade and Lisa Feldman Barrett, the authors state (2):

'*In conclusion, positive emotions can be an important factor that buffers individuals against maladaptive health outcomes. Emerging research indicates that finding ways to cultivate meaningful positive emotions is a critical necessity for optimal physical and psychological functioning. Indeed positive emotions are good for your health. With increasing research, we continue to substantiate empirically age-old folk theories about positive emotions and health that have persisted through time'*

For the Ritual to work I stress a positive mindset is essential. I think of it as creating the right mental enviroment to allow the therapeutic consequences of the Ritual to be delivered.

'Shit happens,'in every life. It is a given. Keeping the mind happy and content is vital. However dark your day, you must include some light. You must bring to your life hobbies, passions, activities, people that nurture you and let in contentment.

Avoid negative people and negative situations. Don't be knocked back by criticism. Human beings are experts at putting others down, don't buy in to adverse comments directed at you or overheard. Take constructive criticism seriously but do not take it personally. Realise many who criticise are malcontented. Many have issues to deal with and the easy way is to take the failings of their own life out on somebody else. The healing way is to listen to yourself, to your heart, to know what is getting in your way, getting you down, and deal with it.

Action, not *in action* is healing. I believe by the time you finish this book you will know when and how to act in your own life to change the things that need changing.

If you find it impossible to alter your mood go out for a walk.

If you live in the centre of the town I suggest you get on a bus or get in to your car and move yourself to the nearest piece of open countryside.

The power of nature is restorative.

Huge vistas and natural landscapes remind us of the power, scale and magnificence of the Universe and the insignificance of ourselves.

If you were not born with an *über* positive personality. If quite reasonably from time to time you are overwhelmed by the stresses and tensions of day to day living, it is hard at first to develop a mindset that holds only the positive within it.

Changing the way that you think, effectively conditioning your thinking to always turn towards the positive, to accept with conviction the way in which you think directly influences your life and your health, is no easy task. It will not be instantly achieved.

You would accept a need for patience, if within your body you were attempting to promote physical change. You would know instinctively if you joined a gym results would not be immediate. With a programme of exercise it would take weeks to see even minimal changes in your physique. A slight loosening of clothes, improvement in posture, a sense of lightness. It would for the unenthusiastic gym attenders take several months for any change to be realised. So be realistic. Do not expect the mind to rotate from black to white, from stressed to relaxed, from determinedly negative to positive within a matter of days.

In buying this book you have decided to change your life. To make space for health and regeneration. You have decided to believe the power of good health rests with you. That the shape of your future rests in your own hands. That is a heavy tome to carry. Don't panic, just stick with the Ritual. Commit to positivity throughout each performance and you will see positive thoughts multiply. Negativity once reversed is more easily reversed time and time again.

If your mindset is not healthy. If you harbour, ugly, resentful, mean or negative thoughts and wish others ill, the Ritual is unlikely to bring you beneficial results.

In earlier times I was a very competitive man, but after a year of performing the Ritual I had a revelation; there is enough to go around. Enough money. Enough food. Enough clothing. Enough unloved human beings with whom to form lasting relationships. Enough work if you are flexible and creative and willing to learn. There is no need, at least if you live in the Western hemisphere, and it is not a matter of life or death, to seek to stand at the front of the queue, for anything.

Be driven by sensible goals. Caring for others. Encouraging those around you. Help someone every day. Strive to have a warm safe place you can call home. It does not matter about its size. It matters about how you feel in it. What your neighbours are like. Success is not money shaped. Indeed all studies in to positive psychology have shown there is no correlate between the amount of money you have and wellbeing. Although giving money to others, developing a sense of altruism, can be good for your health.

Neither is success in life down to material possessions. Your success as a human being does not arrive with a speed boat or a Rolex. Your human success is determined by how you make others feel, by your effort in maximising the good that flows from your time allocated to you on this earth. This, after a lengthy period of engagement with my Rtiual is how I assess success.

What do you, outside of my Ritual experience, think it means to be successful human being? Are you still thinking in terms of those having a designer lifestyle, luxurious living, a London flat, a sea-side retreat, an offshore bank account, a spouse who looks good and a lover who looks even better!

In my opinion you are misguided. Labouring under illusions. Shake them off. Get a life.

Think of what is going on on the inside of your skin.

Think of who you are. What your purpose is on this earth.

If you are here just to accumulate wealth, pause for a

minute and consider the state of your health. How does it seem?

Are you as rich in vigour and energy as you are in euros or sterling?

Is it a fact that you are rich, as your bank account states, or is it the truth you are impoverished. Emotionally and spiritually bankrupt, ill with a continuing unidentifiable malaise? Reduced in real wealth terms by chronic or disabling illness?

Really what good is wealth and a stock pile of assets if your body and every structure within it is paying the price of you living continually on the outside of your existence?

Think of how long, in all probability, according to what the actuaries say, you have left on this earth.

Do the dreaded calculation.

Download or buy or rent from the library a set of actuarial tables that provide average life expectancies. Enter your age in to the calulator.

I tell you what. I will save you time.

I took a look at the Life Expectancy Charts released by the UN Department of Economic and Social Affairs in 2011. The tables set out predicted male and female life expectancy around the world as matters stood in 2010. For men in the UK in 2011, predicted life expectancy was 77.38 years. If a man dies before this age it is in statistical terms a tragedy. If he survives beyond the age it is a blessing.

For women, predicted life expectancy in 2011, was a life of 82.57 years.

Women live longer. It is a fact.

They listen more, pay more attention, are likely to eat a more sensible diet, avoid risk, abuse alcohol and drugs less. They are more receptive to new ideas and alternative healing suggestions, which makes them more likely to perform the Ritual!

If your wife has begun to perform the Ritual, perhaps to close the already evident life expectancy gap, it may be wise to follow her example!

So, let us continue. We know to what age a male or female in the UK is likely to live. Let us move to the part of the calculation that causes the book to fall, the mouth to open, the brain to flinch as the fact of mortality is presented.

Enter your own age now in to the calculator and substract the age you are from the age you are expected to live to and multiply by 365.

A man aged 63 in 2011 can expect to live to the age of 77.38 years, that is for another 14.38 years or for another 5248.7 days.

How many 63 year olds out there would think that was a generous allocation of days that remained?

I bet every male of 63 would like their remaining number of days to be higher.

We are programmed for life. We have an instinct for it. We will claw our way back from death.

I have performed this calculation with numerous people and almost without exception the person confronted with the likely length of the remainder of their life has been jolted out of the indifference, that is usually paid to the average number of days we can all expect to live, towards a sudden and terrifying revelation that life is brief. The numbers are small. We should not waste our days.

Do the calculation for your own life based on your own age and when the number comes out of the calculator consider how you feel.

What is important? To live a healthier more purposeful and engaged life, in an effort to increase the number of days that you will live in good shape? Or the investments you have in the bank and the annual yield from your shares?

What does the almost universal reaction to the, 'life that is left for me', equation, tell us about human beings?

Does it tell us human beings are all greedy or does it tell us, when their attention is drawn to it, human beings are greedy for life?

Let's look at what you are doing with your life.

What kind of energy do you have?

Does life energy flow through and out of you or are there blockages?

Given anything away lately? Something to someone who needed it more? Taken any clothes or shoes or furniture or records or books to a charity shop? Made any charitable donations? Given blood, tissue, a kidney?

Probably not.

Most of us do not give. Most of us hold on tightly to what we have got. Why?

Because when our mindset is unhealthy we live in a Universe inside our heads, in which there is scarcity, where the only energy we know is full of fear that tells us to hoard and hoard and hoard and deny to everyone else what it is we would like for ourselves.

You have to stop this attachment to the feeling of scarcity within yourself. Positive life giving energy is flowing in to you. You cannot stop it; it keeps you alive, it is yours for as long as you live, but if it is not flowing out of you, unrestricted by any blockages, narrowness, enmities, resentments, jealousies, rage, avarice or greed you are making yourself ill. You are damaging your life, ignoring your potential and the fact, that for the sake of yourself, you really have to change.

I am sorry but the Ritual will only work if your internal energy is right. If the environment of yourself is allowing the energy within you to flow.

Your environment is the space you inhabit. The space inside you. The space you take up on earth. The energy filled environment that affects the people around you.

The energy within you has to be right and vital and balanced for the good of your life and your health, and the secret is this, your energy, that is you, can only be the way you should be, if your contained thoughts and emotions are positive, loving and beneficent. Not only towards your family or your dog or your cat, but towards your neighbours and your street and community and town and city and country and continent and world.

Remember writing your address when you were ten years old and you started with your name and then your house number and your road and your city and your country and your continent and your world, ending up with the Universe, the Cosmos, Space? Identifying yourself as a resident of the biggest and emptiest place your mind could encompass. Well in those moments of connectivity with all the energies of the earth your own internal energy, the inner environment I describe, would have been perfect for a performance of the Ritual to begin.

The energy you displayed when writing your cosmic address was magnificent, grandiose, open and unlimited. The possessor of such energy could only ever present as an equally magnificent being.

If something has changed, not your age or your collar or dress size, but something intrinsic to you that means now when you are older you cannot connect with that juvenile expansiveness you must pay attention to what has happened or is happening. The containment of your imagination, your thought and connectivity in a lesser emotionally constrained sphere is not good for your life or your health.

Life events affect the energy we display. Mounting pressures, depression, conflict, stress, a sense of worthlessness, reduce the energy we exude and possess until our ability to connect with the world beyond us and others within it is diminished.

The benefits the Ritual delivers can be maximised when our energy is flowing as it should be and it is positive.

If you feel flat, 'out of sorts', agitated, bitter, angry, it is likely you are not feeling positive. It is probable you are filled with negativity and that any connection between your own being and the positive energy of the Universe has been temporarily suspended. If you are in a depressed emotional state, if there is conflict within you, it is best to consider what has happened in your life and to work it out. What event, happening, circumstance or person has blocked or is blocking the energy of your life? We must identify the problem and if we are to maximise the benefit we obtain from the Ritual we must deal with the identified problem first.

It is part of repairing our mindset. The mind is the director of thought and constructor of emotion, but the mind can only work with the energy of a life. If the energy flowing in to a mind is twisted, constricted or altered by emotional blockages and negativity, to an energy that is malign and damaging to the body it possesses or to others, something has gone awry. Snag of wiring. Nothing serious. Nothing the brain cannot re-wire if things are seen differently. If a mindset is altered from black to white.

We are all wired in the same way. We all have good days and bad days, but the days when we truly live to our full potential are the days in which we are connected to the positive energy of our existence. Every other energy that we generate is, I believe,' off - key'. Disabling in the sense that it does not allow us to be the best that we can be.

To be a healthy functioning human being is to be a charged and positive being. It is what the world requires of us, but before we take on that challenge, the big one, of fixing the planet, let's consider fixing ourselves. Allow only positivity to exist within the space of yourself and the Ritual will deliver quite exceptional results.

If you are not persuaded by my discourse consider this, optimists recover better from medical procedures, such as coronary by-pass surgery, have healthier immune systems and live longer, both in general and when suffering from conditions such as cancer, heart disease and kidney failure. (3)

Research has shown the health benefits of positivity are comparable in importance to the harm done by stress and pessimism. Positivity reduces levels of stress and so levels of cortisol. It is thought positivity may reduce susceptibility to disease by dampening the systematic nervous system, which governs fight or flight responses, and strengthening the para-sympathetic nervous system, which governs, rest and digestion. (4)

Recently analysed data from the Georgia Centenarian Study (5) recognises that a centenarian's feelings about their own health, well-being and support systems, rather than biological measures such as blood pressure and blood sugar, are strong predictors of longevity and survival. My Ritual is right on the bullseye of the target of longevity in promoting a positive assessment of my health, well-being and life in general.

A recent paper which appeared in the Journal of Applied Psychology (6) suggests the evidence, which now exists, associating a positive mindset and enjoyment of life with better health and longer life, is even stronger than the research evidence which links obesity to disease and to premature death. Positivity is the platform upon which longevity is built.

We are explorers remember that. Remember that one day our naive efforts to consider the way that our bodies worked and to unravel the secrets of longevity will be looked at sympathetically by those who may be two hundred years old.

The secrets of longer more empowered living are gradually being revealed by science.

Anthony D.Ong from the Department of Human Development at Cornell University in his paper, *Pathways Linking Positive Emotion and Health In Later Life (7)* tells us that:

'Numerous changes in physiological functioning accompany the ageing process. Gradual declines in fundamental aspects of the neuroendocrine, cardiovascular, and immune systems contribute to increased risks for morbidity and mortality'

Anthony Ong identifies and analyses, '*plausible pathways that may underlie the association between positive emotion and health.*

The firm conclusion drawn is that positivity and health are linked. This is a definite. The reason for the clear association between the two requires further research, but the fact is nevertheless the fact, positivity in itself is life sustaining. Combine positivity with the Ritual and you have a routine that will deliver fantastic results for your life.

_____ CHAPTER TWELVE _____

MIRACLES

*A miracle that's possible for anyone is possible for everyone.
(1)*

One of the most difficult things for anyone engaging with the Ritual to accept is that something so available, so unlicensed, so cheap, could actually work.

We are not programmed to accept that we as individuals, without an intervening medical specialist, or alternative health practitioner, maji or magician, have power over our own health. We are used to seeking advice, to handing over our health care to someone else? The Ritual of abdication has in itself become therapeutic. Once troubled by symptoms, we take part, not in a ritual of my type, but in the ritual of modern healthcare; we receive pills, or potions, or wait as a day patient for some medical procedure or in a hospital for tests upon the body we possess, and at the end of this process, at the culmination of this ritual of intervention, in the majority of instances, our symptoms disappear.

We do not think of self-care. Self cure.

Sometimes it is not an option. Any attempt at self healing or self repair would be inappropriate in the case of extreme trauma, when the ritual of intervention is the immediate and only resource we can possibly entertain; but what about in all the other instances of intractable disease and unattainable medical resolution? Drug failure? Adverse reaction to the drugs we are given? Disappointing medical procedures, disillusionment, chronic illness that refuses to go away? What about all the possibilities short of cure? What of prevention, of maintenance of the body that we have? Why even in these discrete areas do we act as if we believe we have no role to play?

Why do we not once think of attempting to access within our selves something the medical profession cannot gain access to, our own innate ability to heal?

Isn't the truth that the fact of our own ability to care for our body and the systems within it, is something that never even crosses our mind?

Isn't it right most of us know absolutely nothing at all about our body's ability to engage with illness and produce the same results as pills or drugs, because it is something that is never ever revealed to us, talked about, brought to the forefront of education when we talk about health?

Self- healing, self engagement with the resources of healing within us is something that takes us so far beyond that which we are used to our mind does not even begin to entertain it?

We are like the tiny corner shop standing next door to the megalithic superstore. Within our small shop we may have goods of such rarity quality and epicurean delight we could in many ways outstrip the giant we stand in the shadow of, even with all its best bargains and best buying power, but it would never once cross our mind we could compete on equal terms, in an entirely different way.

I believe the vastness and indeed the impressiveness of the latest drug treatments and procedures has blinded the ordinary man or woman to any power they may have within themselves to heal or even prevent the onset of illness; it is quite simply something we never consider.

We have, *en masse*, fallen in to the thrall of modern medicine, seduced by the size and scale of state healthcare, by the variety of treatments and techniques available for 'healing', we have lost belief in our own power.

Who aware of all the spectacle and investment of the state in health would think of healing themselves? It is almost sacrilegious, because health is our religion and every developed country provides within its state edifices the temples and the robed and gowned equivalent of priests.

Modern medicine is an ever advancing, heavily invested in, scenario of drugs and new procedures. New ways of scanning, new ways of operating, new tablets and techniques, new methods of diagnosis, of seeing within, to observe, with machines costing tens of thousands of pounds, the origin and the progression of disease. Where is the room in this wealthy arena of drug sales and profit, for any man to put up his hand and say,

'I have taken back control. For years I have been intervening to create my own health, and it is working. I am healthier than I have ever been, more energized, more ready for my life. My Ritual is the reason.'

What weight of derision would fall upon this man?

What hail of voices in a shower of indignation, outrage and outright scoffing would shout down his preposterous idea? How easy to cast the unconventional in a blinding ridiculous light. How easy to bludgeon life from the bones of a new concept?

Modern healthcare is advanced, I give you that. It is slick and shiny and technological. It is a machine. A vehicle that moves, gathering information with clearer and more perfect diagnostic imagery than any one could ever have imagined. It is a system laden with information and bio-chemicals, with more and more targeted and less invasive procedures, rich in remedies and cures. Why would we not take part? Why would we think of anything else besides booking an appointment and taking our place in the long and winding treatment queue?

Because not every one gets well!

In 2012 8.2 million people died of cancer globally. (2)

Every year, 17.3 million people die globally from cardiovascular disease, with this figure likely to increase to 23.3 million people per annum by 2030. (3)

In 2012 cancer was the most common cause of death in the UK, (registered as the cause of death in 29% of deaths). Circulatory diseases caused the second highest percentage of deaths in the UK in 2012, (cause of death in 28% of registered cases) (4) These figures reveal the vastness of the number of patients in which the outcome of medical intervention is not a cure. They do not reveal, what I consider to be the more interesting and telling detail, of what caused those who did not die to live?

Was it drugs, surgery, science, or was it something else?

If the health service understood every one of us so completely it could make each one of us well whatever our ill, however we presented, I would concede defeat. I would set aside this book and lay myself down to await my fate knowing at the first twinge, at the first moment of weakness, I could present myself to my consultant or GP, accepting it was they who knew my physiology, my psyche, my strengths and vulnerabilities better than I knew them myself and it was they and only they that could make me live as I was intended to live.

In this utopia I would surrender to the scanning techniques, that tell us earlier and with more precision, how ill we are. I would not worry that the very same machines were silent on what had caused my illness to occur. I would accept unquestionably what the medical profession had in store, because if cure were the only possible outcome of surrendering up myself I would be foolish to interfere, to upset the medicinal apple cart, with any homespun engineering, but this is not the position we are in.

It is not known, or it is not perfectly known, what causes the mutation of a cell. It is a matter of medical speculation and debate as to what causes cancer. If it were known in absolute terms there would be no cancers that could not be eradicated. The chilling fact is, it remains a mystery to modern medicine why cancer appears and why in many cases it takes root and is inextinguishable. It is an equal mystery why some who smoke and drink live to an advanced age while others die efficiently in huge numbers, from liver failure and heart disease. Modern medicine deals with everything in analytical terms, it gathers and presents statistics, it is all knowing about incidences and probability, its only real difficulty, its taxing calculation, is in explaining survivors!

The inconsistent, the remarkable, the miraculous who should not, according to the medical men, be alive. Those defiant beings that outlive the predictions and death sentence the medical community hand to them. ' You have two years'. 'You have at best, three months.' 'There is nothing that can be done. I am afraid your disease is terminal. I would suggest you make appropriate arrangements.' 'I would give you a year'.

Twelve years ago I received a phone call from my brother-in-law Peter. He was almost incoherent, tremulous and shaken. As my conversation with him unfolded I managed to understand Peter had been handed his death date by his urology consultant. He had less than two years to live. He was distressed, defeated, and resigned to the forecast delivered to him. He had an aggressive form of prostate cancer that had spread from the prostate to the adjoining lymph glands. There were treatments but little prospect of cure with death likely within a period of two years.

I wanted to punch the consultant who had delivered this news, delivering so emphatically the words that stole hope, that made pointless any positive attack upon disease.

How could a medical professional be allowed to utter the worst as if it were the only reality in the whole medicinal universe? How could a medical expert not know the psychological impact of his words? Why would a consultant not first present the positive? The fact of ongoing medical research, the campaign to defeat cancer, unfolding treatments, the miracles already seen, the fact that Peter may live longer or less, but possibly longer than two years? Why be so specific? Why engage the patient's brain with a truth that the consciousness would store and hold and cling on to and endeavor to act out?

I was furious.

I was already cynical about the construct of medical care and the interface between drug companies and healers. I told Peter there had to be another way; I told him that he could lie down and accept the verdict or give everything he had within himself to begin a fight for his life. I pep talked my brother- in – law out of negativity, into believing in his power to intervene in his own health and then he pep talked himself. Every day. Every day for the last twelve years Peter has been evangelical in his commitment to healing his body by harnessing the resources within him. He is now cancer free. He is a living example of a survivor who simply refused to accept the diagnosis given and began his own campaign.

Peter has thrown everything at his disease. Driven and sustained by his belief that alternative therapies can defeat the cancer that he has, he has tried everything, open mindedly, with optimism and now on scans his cancer cannot be seen. His tumour has not only regressed it has disappeared.

Peter embarked on a mission to live. I persuaded him his cancer could be defeated and he believed me. He embarked on a campaign to heal himself.

He attended the Cambridge Cancer Centre; underwent spiritual healing, connecting whole-heartedly with the process, visualising as instructed, believing, believing, that his cancer was being beaten. He attended a psychic surgeon, believed his tumour had been cut out. He ate apricot kernels believing they were poisonous to cancer cells. He swallowed high doses of vitamin C believing they would enhance his immunity.

He believed in his power to eradicate cancer from his body with such conviction he started helping others to take on their own cancers. He began to counsel and encourage, to deliver talks in hospitals. His mindset changed from vulnerable to invincible.

A year after his diagnosis Peter had an MRI scan at the Royal Hammersmith hospital in London. His lymph glands were clear of cancer cells and the tumour in the prostate had significantly regressed. A different consultant to that handing out the original diagnosis expressed delight and a good degree of amazement when comparing this second Hammersmith scan with the first made available from the first hospital at which the original diagnosis of cancer had been made.

I have used the term evangelical. No other will suffice. Peter became a shining beacon of belief. On reflection, knowing what I know now after researching for this book, it is possible Peter created multiple placebo effects, as he imbibed his vitamin C drinks, chewed on his apricot kernels, felt the heat of spiritual and psychic energy, setting off a chain reaction of healing within himself.

From a day or so after his diagnosis until this very day Peter has demonstrated an absolute and unshakeable belief in his body's power to heal itself.

The strength of Peter's belief in his inner reserves has led him to therapies he would never have considered. Peter accepted the drugs he was offered by the medical profession. The drugs would have given him his two allocated years but without his approach of confronting his disease through confronting himself and harnessing the resources of his own immune system and his innate ability to intervene in his wellbeing to deliver his own health he would not, I firmly believe, have received his further decade.

Peter's experience compounds my belief in the need for my daily Ritual. However impressive our current system of conventional medical care, however great the investment of a country in its health service there is always room I consider for the form of self communication and self intervention that my Ritual provides.

We are, every cell of ourselves. We are unique. We can profit from everything this century provides in terms of modern pills and modern techniques but if at some point we do not recognise it is more complicated than that, that each of us, every single human being on this earth, carries within themselves the gift of longevity and health, we will die having only partially lived, and nothing in science will save us from the tragedy of those facts.

To recognise that we have a responsibility for our health and well being, that we are not powerless, is to accept that we can perform miracles. That is hard for any one of us who has lived according to the constructs of paternalistic government and medicine to entertain.

We are used to public health guidance, delivered with every good intention, telling us how much alcohol we can drink, not to smoke, what to eat, telling us whether fats or fruit or both are good or bad for our health. We entertain the vacillations in advice, accept the differing suggestions and act upon them unknowing that in the back- ground of our lives scientists in contest for funds and acclaim are constantly changing their minds. (5)

We feel ill and we seek a pill. We feel ill for long enough and we seek a procedure. We swallow in good faith chemicals that trigger molecular reactions as powerful as tsunami's upon our sensitive systems without regard to side effects, or consequences of system imploding upon system. We are believers, but we may be believing in the wrong things. A pill may cure an ill but cause imbalance elsewhere. A procedure may make matters worse not better. We are gullible, entranced. We are used to being told by others how not to be ill. It is, I agree, a truly shattering and terrifying prospect to consider we can be in charge of our own maintenance and repair, to be told we can go it alone.

It is terrifying but it is correct. We cannot live forever, not yet, but we can live longer in better health, with greater energy drive and capability, by intervening in our own being, than we can achieve by simply holding out our hand and saying to those ready to administer to us, 'give me the latest pill'.

CHANGE OF PERSPECTIVE

This chapter is about miracles. To engage with my Ritual in an effective way a mindset that entertains miracles is a necessity. The biggest miracle of all is inside the body you possess. You are a walking miracle. Entertain that fact. Let it permeate your consciousness; you are the unrealised miracle of yourself.

It is time to start paying attention to the absolutely unrepeatable marvel of your own life. You are unique but your engineering is human standard. You have within yourself 100 trillion cells. 300 million of these cells die and are replaced every minute that you live. You have a heart that beats up to 100, 000 times every day. 60,000 miles of blood vessels form the carriageway of your blood. Your eye blinks on average 6 million times in a year. (6). This is the astounding human form, that is robust enough to survive for around 100 years. Isn't that miraculous?

Twenty thousand recorded diseases affect the human body in twenty thousand different ways. That is a recorded twenty thousand attempts of assault upon a grouping of 100 trillion cells, each group modified by individual genetics to form an individual, who although engineered in the same way as every other human being on earth, is absolutely and wonderfully, unique. Imagine the bio - chemist who could come up with a formula to intervene in such staggering mathematics! The genius of the scientist required to invent a pill so perfect it could intervene to deliver healing across multiple trillions of permutations of life. Bam! One tablet, one procedure, the bullseye of healing every time.

Reflect upon the intelligence required for that and then ask your self how complex is the formula of healing and health? Who or what is likely to possess the code to heal, maintain and repair every person on this earth? Is it likely, do you think, that the secret of individual wellness lies externally to ourselves or within us? Where would you, if you had the power to create a human being, safely put the key to longevity?

I believe, without doubt, as the man on the night- club door told me when I was very much younger than I am now, all we need for life is inside us. The secret to maintaining our body in good shape is ours to access.

I believe we can maintain and repair the body that we have by reversing our thinking, accepting responsibility and working every day to commune with, encourage and inspire, the systems that we rely upon. Endocrine, cardiovascular, circulatory, immune, digestive, lymphatic, they can all be stimulated to work as well as they have ever done, free of all disease, if we believe wellness is the inevitable consequence of the daily ritual we perform.

It is all about belief.

And there we have it. We have come full circle. We are almost at the end of this book of introduction to my Ritual technique and we are back to the act of belief.

To believe in the almost magical, in something more powerful than all of contemporary science is an almost impossible thing, but it can be done, and it is in the doing, in this act of believing that we access our own gift to preserve and restore the body that we have. Open and complete acceptance of our own potential to orchestrate our health is the basis upon which my Ritual works and the key to obtaining every described result.

As I write this chapter I am able only to hold up my own life as example of the power my Ritual has, because, at the beginning of this quest to share what has happened in my own life I am my Ritual's only disciple. Slim evidence I know upon which to build conviction and belief in others but I have help from elsewhere.

There is in human history astounding evidence of events of human healing and spontaneous remission from the very worst of diseases, including cancer, that defy the medical men; that throw science and conventional medicine in to disarray quite simply because the documented events occurred beyond the boundaries of science. The cases I present are in scientific terms, in terms of what is known about the body, the immune system and human resistance to disease, inexplicable. They are events so far from the expected, so far at the limits of human and medical credence that they are defined as miraculous.

If by the end of this chapter you are prepared to believe in miracles I will be delighted. Not simply because you will have engaged with and have been persuaded by the facts I have collated but because you will then have the mindset, the open mindedness needed for my Ritual to begin to do its work.

MODERN DAY MIRACLES

Belief cures. Any good Catholic will tell you that. The most virulent and disabling of conditions inflicted upon a human being have been eradicated by acts of faith. The cases are documented, verified and authenticated. Really! It is an astounding fact that there is available to mankind a record of miracles, which should we wish to do so, we can sit down and consider at any time.

The record, I am writing about, is maintained by the Lourdes Medical Bureau. The function of this unlikely organisation is to transfer medical investigation of apparent cures associated with the shrine within the Sanctuary of Our Lady of Lourdes to the International Medical Committee of Lourdes. The committee investigate every aspect of a purported 'cure' to see if it can be categorised as medically inexplicable.

For a cure to be recognised, the original diagnosis of disability or illness afflicting the person cured must be verified by inspection of medical records. The suffered affliction must be regarded as incurable by means available to medicine at the time the cure occurred. The cure must happen in Lourdes or within the vicinity of the shrine. The cure must be immediate, providing rapid resolution of symptoms and signs of illness. The cure must be complete, leaving no residual impairment, and if all of that were not enough, at the time a 'cure' is recognised by the committee, it must be capable of being considered a cure that is permanent.

Between 1858 and 2013, thousands of instances of alleged 'cure' have been investigated by the committee; that is not so remarkable as people visit Lourdes from all over the world and bathe and drink the waters from the shrine in the hope that the Lady of Lourdes will intervene in their condition to heal them. What is remarkable is that 67 truly astounding instances of 'cure' have been investigated and considered to meet all of the criteria I set out above.

In each of the 67 cases verified by the committee, the disability removed, was according to the assessment made by modern medicine, medically incurable at the time the cure was delivered. Which means if the 67 people now regarded as the recipients of a miracle had not sought some other route beyond the conventional, beyond the walls and corridors of contemporary medicine, they would, each of them, have lived out their life in misery and pain.

I suggest you read the entire record of miracles recorded by the Bureau. It is inappropriate for me to recite here the entire record of those healed. I highlight the cases that have had the greatest impact upon my own mind. I begin with the case of Serge Perrin from Lion'd'Angers in France. This case moved me because I have a background in optics. I was in another life a practising optician and I realise from my own medical training that the miracle of Serge Perrin's cure is not just improbable but impossible in terms of what is known of the biology of the human eye.

Serge Perrin visited Lourdes on the 1st May 1970. At the time of his visit to the shrine Serge Perrin was 41 years old. From the age of 35 he had suffered recurrent right hemiplegia, with ocular lesions, due to bilateral carotid artery disorders. By October 1969 Serge Perrin had been granted a level 3 invalidity pension in France as he was able to do nothing alone. The Neurological Unit in the Hospital at Rennes had decided surgical intervention was pointless and Serge Perrin was left to face a future of increasing disability and despair. At the time of his visit to Lourdes in 1970 he was partially paralysed on the right side and unable to walk. He retained some residual sight but was considered almost blind in both eyes. He presented at Lourdes as an incurable invalid with a prognosis for further decline.

On the 1st May 1970 Serge Perrin attended the ceremony of the anointing of the sick by the waters of the Shrine. It is reported that during the ceremony Serge Perrin began to feel sensation return in his paralysed limbs. In the afternoon he felt he could walk, rising from his wheelchair and refusing the aid of walking sticks he moved independently for the first time in years. Most wonderfully he could see, perfectly, without the aid of the very thick spectacles he had relied upon to provide him with some outline imagery. From 1964 he had suffered with a loss of vision but within hours of the ceremony at Lourdes his full sight was restored.

Upon his return home he was assessed in the hospital at Rennes and medically there was nothing to be seen. He was no longer disabled. Objectively he was cured but the process of verification of his cure, to the point of acceptance by the medical profession took another six years. It was in 1976, on the joint report of a neurologist, Professor Mouren, and an ophthalmologist, Dr Bartoli, that the Medical Committee of Lourdes, in a somewhat half- hearted acceptance of the miracle recorded;

'The cure of this condition can be considered as happening in a most unusual way from the medical point of view'.

On the 24th December 1976, a young girl Delizia Cirolli from Sicily was taken to Lourdes by her parents. Delizia suffered a Ewing's sarcoma of the right knee and was facing amputation of her lower right leg. Her mother refused to allow her to be amputated upon and took her to Lourdes instead. After this visit to Lourdes the tumour on her knee began to regress. The regression was rapid until almost no evidence of the tumour remained. The disappearance of the tumour left the right tibia angulated. An operation was required to correct the angulation, which was successful. The right leg grew normally after this surgical intervention. Delizia's cure was recognised on the 2th June 1989. (7)

These two examples strike me as compelling because they do not obviously present as examples of belief of the person cured believing in the Virgin. It was others in their lives that believed. In the case of Serge Perrin it was his wife, in the case of Delizia it was her mother. Did wife and mother believe with such conviction in a future without disability in it for husband and for daughter that the minds of the latter were also persuaded? Was it deity or belief that intervened at the Shrine? I would not presume to know. It is enough for me to believe in miracles. To know whatever the limits of surgery and drugs we can always turn elsewhere. The chemical potency of belief is, I consider, never to be underplayed.

SPONTANEOUS REMISSION OF CANCER

What is that?

It is a cure in which a deity is never implicated. It is the amazing reaction of the body when hope is lost, to suddenly begin to respond to the destruction of disease that has caused the devastation of cells and systems, to reverse that destruction, obliterating it, restoring health within the body until cancer or other illness can be said to have 'gone', 'disappeared', 'regressed'.

In 1993, the Institute of Noetic Sciences, (An institute dedicated to expanding science beyond conventional paradigms), published, *Spontaneous Remission: An Annotated Bibliography*. In this work the authors, Caryle Hirschberg and Brendan O'Regan define spontaneous remission as,

'the disappearance, complete or incomplete, of a disease or cancer without medical treatment or treatment that is considered inadequate to produce the resulting disappearance of the disease or tumor'.

Hirschberg and O'Regan document 3500 instances of spontaneous remission within 800 medical and other journals across 20 languages, with reporting of the event of remission only increasing in recent decades.

We make nothing of the circumstance of spontaneous remission of disease because it is not routinely brought to our attention. If hope matters to healing a human being, and past testimonies suggest that it does, (8) should we not know that in thousands of cases of hopelessness, of life slipping beyond the bounds of medical restoration, plenty of people have lived?

If we knew that our body and mind could and frequently do perform in unexpected ways would it not compound our belief in ourselves? If belief really does fire the mind to engage the body in spectacular ways may not remission become a norm if belief could be harnessed? If indeed the essence of the placebo response could be learned and taught, what would health look like then?

I believe we are at the beginning of understanding that the limits of our life are well beyond those set by contemporary medical science. My Ritual demonstrates to me the vast resources and potential within us that remain to be harnessed.

I consider it a great wrong that investment continues to be principally in bio-chemicals, in adjusting molecular structure and reaction rather than in understanding mind-body interaction. I am powerless. I can do nothing about the pharmaceutical giants or the ambition they have but I can draw attention to the facts that remain in the shadows. We are far more powerful, resourceful and complex than medical textbooks of anatomy and neurobiology allow.

I believe miracles occur, disease vanishes, when we access within ourselves, something presently beyond medical understanding. *Ronald Peters, MD, MPH, (9)* in his paper on the Spontaneous Remission of Cancer looks at factors those experiencing a sudden and spontaneous and long- term remission of their disease have in common. Prior to commencing an analysis of common factors he quotes Dr. Fred Stewart, an American pathologist who in 1952, in a speech delivered at the University of Texas MD Anderson Hospital stated the following;

'Thinking in the cancer field is perhaps too largely directed to methods of artificial destruction of the cancer cell either by its radical removal or its chemical destruction. There has not been enough thought given to biological control by the host'

I find this statement both heartening and depressing. It is uplifting that several decades ago the part a human had to play in his or her own disease was discussed at a medical conference. It is a fact to induce despair that over the course of sixty years investment has not been made in finding out just how much control each of us as 'biological host' has in the prevention, creation or eradication of our illness.

Ronald Peters concludes that the consciousness of the patient has a role to play in spontaneous remission. He writes:

'Because modern medicine is mostly governed by the molecular medicine paradigm, most doctors try to explain the phenomenon of remission by changes in the immune system and not changes in consciousness.' .....'...the majority of research into the remission of disease is devoted to biochemical and immunological mechanisms and not in to the mechanisms of consciousness, or, the attitudinal, emotional, social and other psychological experiences that were part of the remission and may strongly influence immunity through yet to be discovered mechanisms.'(10)

Within his paper Ronald Peters produces an action plan for those facing cancer. He prefaces his proposed treatment plan with the following statement. When reading it I ask you to remember he is writing as a trained member of the medical profession, but with I feel, considerably more insight than the majority of prescribers.

'*In the future doctors will recognize the unity of mind and body, as well as the enormous wisdom and natural healing power that is built into us all. While it is too early to explain the psychophysiology of spontaneous remission, we know enough to take action to increase the chances of recovery*'

Ronald Peters proposes a collection of measures a patient can take to promote a remission from cancer, from changing diet, to practising meditation, to taking responsibility for the disease, expressing emotions and releasing dysfunctional beliefs, to taking supplements.

Dr Peters brings miracles within the grasp of anyone who is ill, by bringing miracles closer, away from the celestial to the everyday. His suggestions for inducing what has always been regarded as miraculous, the sudden and spontaneous remission of a virulent and devastating disease process, recognises the potential, an individual has, to play a part in the drama of a terminal diagnosis, to steer the body away from death to life.

We can create the miracle. I am saying no more than that. Miracles happen, they happen every day, but for a reason that is not clear to me, they are not broadcast, reported as headline news, included before the weather forecast to awaken belief and bring the possibility of self -healing to the forefront of individual consciousness.

—————— CHAPTER THIRTEEN ——————

DIET AND LIFESTYLE

WHY LIFE GOALS ARE IMPORTANT AND COUNTING CALORIES PROBABLY IS NOT

DIET

It is important that we have a good relationship with the food that we eat. I am serious about that. When you sit down to dinner you are on a date, not only with your family or the person in front of you but also with your food. Appreciate the food that you eat, recognise the flavour in it, the power that it has within it to do the body good and the brain. Choose your food well. After all it has an enormous job to do.

And let us get this straight, right at the beginning of this chapter full of the best advice I can give to you based upon my own life experience, eating well does not mean paying a lot for your food. Infact some of the worst, and indeed the most ludicrous, wildly over priced, dinners, I have eaten have been served to me in some of the best restaurants on earth. Some of the best, most flavoursome, nutritious meals of my existence have been the cheapest. I remember eating sardines on a quayside in Portugal at one euro a plate and knowing I would carry the flavor and the temptation of the smell of the freshly grilled fish with me all of my life.

I have just now considered the websites of three leading supermarkets. Which ever I chose I found I could buy enough white fish, vegetables and potatoes, to feed a family of four for just over £4.35. If I threw in some mixed herbs to flavour the fish my meal would still cost under a fiver.

But do not think I am in the business of creating menus, I am not. If McDonalds or Burger King serve up the kind of food that delights your palette my advice to you is go ahead and stand in their queues. It is in my opinion a toxic, excessive, remote from your self, life style, that is bad for you not hamburgers.

But let's get back to the essence of my advice to you on diet.

Eat simply, eat wisely, eat as well as you can, that is what I think you should do, respect your self and your food.

Do you consider you are respecting your body and your mind when you choose a greasy take away or a snatched, already two day old, packaged ready meal for your evening meal? Or are you simply not engaging with the relationship you should have with the food you place in to your mouth?

Quick fix meals flung down on the counter top, or food in boxes prepared by strangers in some remote food processing plant give only one message to the mind. Nurturing the body is a casual affair. Anything will suffice. If the mind gets the message that fuelling and maintaining the blood, bone and fibre of the body is of secondary importance, something others take care of, what good do you think you do to your self. Mind body communication is dramatically important. The early chapters of this book are intended to demonstrate that.

Think about what you are eating that is all I am asking you to do.

You will see from the details I provide of my own diet, no elaborate preparation of meals is required, in fact the converse, the simpler, less complicated and less over worked the routines of preparation, the more I believe my food will do me good.

These are my rules for healthy eating.
1. Eat what ever you like, but eat little of it and eat often.
2. Feel good about those things you choose to eat and drink and as you place them in to your mouth relish the individual flavours in the food you have chosen. Feel grateful for the food and drink you are provided with.
3. Eat mindfully with concentration and appreciation. As you chew or swallow believe in the power the food and drink you are consuming has within it to sustain you and furnish you with good health.
4. Focus on the connection between the food you are eating and the drink you are drinking and the task in hand of providing nutrition to your body and to your mind.
5. Believe in your food. Believe it is doing you good and if it is not bleach or a block of chemical toxins it probably will be.

That's it; those are the rules!

No boundaries pre supposed between the healthy and the un –healthy ingredient. No list supplied of things to avoid, things to add in or take out, products to increase or reduce. That is for other books, for other experts. I am not a dietician. I am an ordinary man living well and longer I believe, than I other wise would, as a result of imposing a new set of rules upon my self. This book is about the Ritual of my life and eating as I do supplements the Ritual I perform.

In simple terms, although I have provided what I label my 'rules' for eating well, I would urge everyone to think for themselves, to work with their own instinct and create their own rules, which direct them, to eat for their own health.

Living longer requires a certain level of nutrition, of hydration, that's obvious, but it requires much more than that, it requires us to change the relationship we have with our food and most fundamentally our view of the consequences of eating and drinking as we do?

Do we believe what we have chosen is good for us or are we burdened by guilt? Are we eating and drinking at cross-purposes with our underlying instinct that sends a very clear message to our brain that certain things we are prone to eat and drink are likely to do us harm?

For our food and drink to sustain us, to preserve the elasticity in our tissues, the strength in our bones, the life in our cells, we have to believe every bite and sip that we take is building our health, promoting our longevity, creating the energy we possess. We have to know this profoundly, deep within our consciousness. If we believe in our diet as I describe, I am certain the body responds. I have witnessed this for myself within my own life. I have no doubt each of us will live longer, in better shape, if we believe as we eat and drink, our food is doing us good.

It is the edible placebo effect!

It is in my opinion the connection between our thoughts and our diets that matter, not the differing constituent elements of each diet that exists on the face of this earth.

Consider the randomness of the diets upon our planet. Those in the East consumed with a passion for the raw, the unadulterated sushi of the Japanese, Mexico on fire with chillies in every dish. Mongolia in love with boiled mutton and marmot, an entire nation subsisting on a diet ill advised in the West, 100% animal protein and fat.

The exact nature of what we put in to our mouth does not appear to matter a great deal. Our emotional and intellectual relationship with our food, I believe does, and I propose it matters 100%.

John Robbins in his wonderfully inspiring book, *Healthy at 100* (1) is one of the authors I respect to provide me with some useful insights about diet. His study of the diet of the peoples of Abkhasian in the Caucasus south of Russia, the Vilcabamba in the South America Andes, and the Hunzans in Central Asia, purportedly three groups demonstrating the greatest longevity on earth, (not only living for the greatest period of chronological time) but in great shape, free of disease and with maintained vitality, leads him to write this (2):

'It is actually quite intriguing how similar the typical Hunzan diet is to the traditional diets of the Vilcabambans and the Abkhasians. Though they live in very different parts of the world, the traditional diets of all three of these extraordinarily healthy societies are very low in calories by modern standards. In all three cases, protein and fat are almost entirely of vegetable origin. And all three depend on natural foods, rather than processed and manufactured ones'.

John Robbins describes Abkhasians eating a ' salad of green vegetables freshly picked from the garden for breakfast', the exact nature of the salad varying with the seasons. Each meal being accompanied by a cornmeal porridge. He tells us of the lack of knowledge the Vilcabamba have of processed foods or preservatives and of the passion the Hunzas have for fruit. Perhaps those urging us to flee from fruit sugar should take note of his words;

Of the Hunza diet, John Robbins writes:

'What kind of food do the Hunzas grow on the fertile terraces that have been called one of the great wonders of the world? They grow a wide variety of fruit, including apricots, peaches, pears, apples, plums, grapes, cherries, mulberries, figs, and many types of melons. They enjoy all these plus a multitude of wild berries, both fresh and sun-dried. Their

apples are huge, weighing more than a pound each. But of all their fruits, the ones they eat by far the most are their celebrated apricots.'

'No where in his treatise on longevity does John Robbins mention the emotional relationship the Hunzas, the Abkhasians, or the Vilcabamba have with their food. He talks of the structure of the societies, the respect for the aged and for the wisdom of the aged. He describes the vast amounts of exercise taken naturally day- by -day and notes the freshness and the lack of adulteration of food in the three diets. Beyond this he does not go. He certainly never mentions an edible placebo response but to me all three peoples in their approach to their nutrition, pay attention, seek out flavour, grow fresh, the fruit and vegetables they place upon their plate. It seems to me inevitable that each of these diverse peoples believe as they consume the food they have produced it is doing them good. They after all have the lessons of their forbears to draw upon. They have witnessed the ritual of their lives deliver ages of 120 and beyond. Why would they not believe that in every bite of their diet longevity lies.

Moreover these peoples from three very different ethnic groupings appear to relish the collection and production of their food. Consider the joy of developing yet another variety of apricot, of hunting for and consuming the freshest berries. Eating amongst each of these peoples appears a celebration, a harvesting of the earth. Changing ingredients to match the seasons, eating what the earth provides. What stark contrast their routines provide with the irritation of crowded supermarkets and check out queues.

The greatest distinction between our overloaded packaged ready meal life style and these peoples in some of the remotest locations on Earth, is, in my opinion, that they, in contrast to us, never fail to pay attention. Never fail to communicate to the mind that nurturing the body through the preparation of food is a ritual worthy of great respect, dedication and effort. It seems to me inevitable, if, as I suggest, the body responds to information and messages delivered to the brain, that each of these peoples has the position just right. They are, I suggest, living the consequences of digesting an edible placebo.

I have Italian friends living in the North of Italy who live in the same way. They know the month to eat grapes, the month for strawberries, the month for pomegranates. When I suggest I can eat each of these fruits all year round simply by going to the supermarket they consider me as if I am not fully formed, as If I have not one clue about how to truly live. It is to them as if I am simply eating for the sake of it rather than eating in tune with the seasons as nature intends, to nurture the body I possess.

If we don't enjoy what we eat, have no belief in the power of our food to sustain us and instead feel constant dissatisfaction, hunger, or the converse a burdensome guilt from over indulgence, a sluggishness from consumption of excess sugar and fats, how can we expect beneficial results? How can we expect our body to thrive?

Pay attention. If you have enough money to feed yourself and to have a choice in what goes in to the shopping basket. Pay attention. That is all that is required to suddenly and without substantial effort open the channels of communication between brain and mind and between mind and body.

If you perform the Ritual and are prepared to eat for your health rather than for a troubled psyche or wildly out of control ego you will begin to see your body be what it is supposed to be. You will begin to recover the form nature intended for you. You will not be on a diet you will be inside your diet, creator of it, taker of it, and gainer from it. You will be feeding your body what is needed for your life cutting out all that serves no purpose and is unnecessary. All the blurring messages that result not from what your body needs but from an over layering of emotional messaging that can only conflict with the edible placebo will cease.

When you begin to make every bite count in the conversation you are having with yourself I have no doubt your mind will believe in only beneficial consequences resulting from the food you put in to your mouth and the body will reap the benefits of the changes that have been made.

I would stress there is no need to remove either pleasure or taste when choosing the foods you decide to consume. As my 98 year old mother would tell us, 'a little bit of what you fancy does you good'. Freda includes within her diet a wide variety of what most dieticians would I am sure consider bad and sinful choices! Lard on bread, whiskey in her tea, chocolate gingers. Freda believes each one of these things is good for her, as is boiled beetroot, and a little slice of egg custard!

Freda boils the beetroot she consumes; often she grows it herself. She bakes her egg custard. My mother has lived her life paying attention to her diet. She has paid attention and most importantly she has never eaten to excess. Small portions frequent meals. Freda will eat breakfast, a snack at mid morning, lunch, a snack in the afternoon, an evening meal, something before bed but never an overloaded plate, and almost nothing processed.

Most importantly Freda believes she is eating for her health. She has made the connection. She unknowingly for decades has swallowed the edible placebo and it appears to have worked. She is in annoying and challenging good health, vital and alert. Mentally sharp with views on stocks and shares and how I should live my life. You get the picture I am sure!

Health is in many respects karmic. You cannot be an abuser of yourself, the planet, or those around you and expect to live well. You cannot have a mind at peace with itself capable of maximizing the potential the body has if you are piling in the chemicals and the toxic. If your food comes to you along a trail of exploitation, under payment, ill deserved profit, and you are aware of these things, the emotion your food engenders in you cannot be good. Indifference will not save you; for in my opinion to be nurtured by your diet you must be mindful, aware, appreciative as you eat, of not only the food but of its provenance, of the richness or deprivation in its supply, in the good that it does not only to your life but to the life of the suppliers.

If this is all too big a concept for you to entertain, fix yourself on Chapter Five, perform the Ritual, alter your mind set, see yourself inside and out, and see yourself as connected not apart. The Ritual alters everything in a very particular way, if you read this page with derision considering you could never live in this way, never pay such attention to something as simple as food, and even more remote and irrelevant to your present life, the consequences for others of the food with which you are provided, stay with me, one future day, further in to your Ritual experience, you will understand why it is necessary to change your perception of the world in which you live.

I know the foods that content my mind.

I later in this chapter provide a map of my eating week so the curious may know the foods that sustain me.

I am guided in my selection of food by my instinct and my upbringing.

A daily performance of the Ritual really does shift perspective. I now see my body from the inside as well as from the outside. I eat oily fish believing it is good for my joints and my heart. It is as if I am looking under the bonnet of a car and considering what oil, grease, or washer fluid may make things run efficiently. Bizarre I know but at least I am paying attention.

I personally would not think of devouring a mountain of cake. I consider the work involved in digesting sugar and fat, the sluggishness with which the machine of myself would run, while all that work of digestion took place. The natural consequence of such a thought pattern is that I simply do not want to choose cake. I choose a handful of almonds instead.

I am boringly moderate in my drinking. In terms of my mechanical imagery drink is an acid harmful to the metal of my working parts. I drink little and if I drink at all I drink the best wine I can afford. I choose soft, fruity wines and I drink an occasional glass. The word on the street is red wine is full of anti-oxidants, the decider for me, in my decision to include a glass of wine within my daily diet is that good red wine is pleasurable. It tastes good, with food it tastes even better and so does the food. Eating if at all possible, should always be pleasurable. That is not always possible but if you have a choice try to make each meal in to a ritual of nutrition, a contemplative act, an act of communication between your body and your mind.

One principal rule I think should be followed is this. I believe each one of us should rid our life of excess and over indulgence. Begin instead to savour flavour. Savour the experience of eating just one square of rich 70% cocoa chocolate. Taste the sensation of the chocolate square melting on to the tongue. When eating becomes an act of appreciation, of nurture, the pattern of eating changes. Inexplicably over eating ends and a new routine begins of supplying the body with the fuel that it needs. It is as if we finally recognise there is a purpose to eating. It is about the body, not the whirlwind of emotions in the mind. It is not about cravings or addiction, it is about sending to our bones, blood, organs, muscles and nerves what they need to function optimally.

The irony is this, the act of paying attention to the food that we eat and the drink that we choose puts an end to the silence. The conversation between mind and body begins. The attention of the mind is directed away from emotional turmoil or other negative forces that drive poor eating choices to the real job in hand, giving the body what it needs to survive and flourish and survive and flourish and survive.

When the mind is concentrated in this way, there is no point to excess, there is point to just enough, to precisely what is needed and no more. Any other motivation or impulse that may drive a person to snatch a high calorie but low in nutrient snack or eat twelve packets of crisps instead of a handful of crisps from one packet is silenced.

Gorging on food is a disconnected action performed on automatic pilot, as is binge drinking. There is no point in the act in itself, no point to the thousands of calories consumed or the oblivion created as the brain is over whelmed by alcohol and the senses disorientated. Over eating, over drinking, has nothing at all to do with nutrition or hydration and everything to do with a person's detachment from themselves. To eat well the mind body connection must be brought to the foreground of a life.

I will say it again; eating well is not about wealth it is about paying attention and making the best choices for your health from the food and drink that is available to you in your life.

MY EATING WEEK

	BREAKFAST	SNACK	LUNCH	SNACK	DINNER
MONDAY	Porridge with oat milk & cinnamon. 1 Poached egg on granary toast. Green Tea with sliced ginger & ½ tsp of turmeric	Banana Green Tea	Small tin of sardines and ½ tin of baked beans on two slices of granary toast. Green Tea	Green Tea 6 small pieces of 70% cocoa chocolate	Starter. Fried fish roe on granary toast. Main. Portion of roast chicken. Root veg mash. Broccoli & green beans. To Drink. Ginger wine diluted in water. Camomile Tea.
TUESDAY	Porridge as Mon. 1 large poached tomato on toast. Green Tea.	Coffee with molasses. Piece of fruit.	Chicken Stew. (Chicken carcass boiled for stock and removed. Chicken pieces. Potatoes. Swede. Parsnips. Carrots. Onion. Butterbeans.) Green Tea.	Mint Tea. 1 Sugar.	Chinese Takeaway. Wandering dragon. (Prepared at my instruction without monosodium glutamate or sauce. Wok fried dry mix of chicken, prawns, duck, carrots, onion, water chestnuts, ginger) Camomile Tea

	BREAKFAST	SNACK	LUNCH	SNACK	DINNER
WEDNESDAY	Porridge with freshly sliced mango. 1 Poached egg on toast. Green Tea	Green Tea. Handful of almonds. Several pieces of 70% cocoa chocolate	Sardines on granary toast with beans. Green Tea	Mint Tea Banana	Grilled 8oz rib eye steak with new potatoes, carrots and broccoli. Camomile Tea.
THURSDAY	Porridge as Wed. Poached egg on toast. Green Tea	Café latte Banana	3 slices of grilled cheese on toast with fresh beetroot. Green Tea	Mint Tea	Indian Restaurant Meal. King prawn on puri. 1/2 main course, King Prawn Saag and 1/2 side dish of Talka Dhal. No rice. One small piece of naan bread. Glass of red wine. Water. Camomile Tea.
FRIDAY	Porridge etc. Boiled egg. Granary Toast. Green tea.	Café latte. Banana.	Small quiche with salad. Earl Grey Tea.	Tea with small portion of cake or fruit tart.	Freshly grilled plaice. Air fried chips. Fruit. 1 glass of white wine. Six or seven squares of 70% cocoa chocolate. Camomile Tea.
SATURDAY	2 slices of grilled back bacon. 1 fried egg. Grilled mushrooms. Granary toast.	Café latte	4" raw black pudding. Prawns with salad. Small bowl of vegetable soup.	Earl Grey Tea. 2 Biscuits.	Seared scallops with salad. Grilled lemon sole, with air fried chips & broccoli. 1 Glass of red wine. Camomile Tea

A friend of mine on reading the lists set out above expressed the following opinion.

'That is the most boring diet on earth. I could not contemplate eating it. I would die of boredom in a fortnight'.

It is absolutely fine for anyone reading this book to think the same. The information I give to you about the foods and beverages I live upon is not meant to be prescriptive. Just as the Ritual is not prescriptive. Every one reading this book must create their own diet, the one that works for their own life. The one that satisfies their palette and meets their tastes. Millions of diverse diets to support a million tailored versions of the Ritual will result. I know this. I know also, the one thing anyone following my advice will achieve is communication with the body that is being fed.

The act of choosing foods that do not conflict with your instinct about their nature or the level of each that should be consumed will change the usual messages held in the brain and mind body communication will proceed along different lines.

I imagine few if any of the diets created by those reading this book will perfectly satisfy the strictures of dieticians. You will see there are plenty of things in my own diet a dietician may object to. Takeaways, outings to an Indian restaurant. Tinned beans, (inevitably processed). Shop purchased biscuits, inevitably full of preservatives, chocolate, even cake. But note this, there is not a lot of any one thing, not a lot of processed and not a lot of protein or fat. Small portions and lots of them, eaten only a handful of hours apart. My eating mantra, eat little, eat often, eat as well as you can, most importantly, eat for yourself.

You are the expert, eat for your tastes, satisfy your palette, indulge yourself. Believe your diet is serving your body, believe in it, know it is doing you good and if, never once, there is an indication from your instinct, your brain messanger, alerting you to toxins and harm, your diet as invented by you, the adult, to your own individual requirements is likely to serve you well.

Ultimately as with all things written about in this book it is down to your belief. It is as simple as convincing yourself that the things you feed upon are doing you good. If you act in this way, rejecting the products and substances you cannot believe in because your instinct intervenes to alert you to potential harm I really do believe you cannot go far wrong.

LIFE GOALS AND PURPOSE IN YOUR LIFE

Essential. The most important aspect of your life. If you want to survive for a very long time. Do something. Create something. If not for yourself for others. Do not sit around bored. Inactivity leads to illness depression and early death. We are programmed to thrive on goals. Set yourself some.

Everyone can do this. Finding a purpose in your life has absolutely nothing to do with money or wealth. Indeed some of the most wasted purposeless lives are led by the indulgent rich. Particularly, by the second and third generation rich, the spenders of wealth created by others.

Money is not needed to create purpose in your life. Getting up from the settee, turning off the television and thinking what you as a human being can achieve over the span of your lifetime is the one essential ingredient to seeking out the reason you are here.

What is your life about?

What is intended?

Are you an educator? Mediator? Do you want to change the world through political intervention or do you want to bake the lightest sponge cake the world has ever eaten? Perhaps you are a geographer and you can not die before you have mapped and understood the dimensions and currents within all the great rivers of the earth. Some cannot die content without having seen the pyramids or the Taj Mahal. Others never leave their garden, wanting only one thing, to win three times in a row the prize for best dahlias, collerette variety.

Whether it is shire horses, corporate enterprise, painting, dentistry, eradication of illness, raising children, life purpose is akin to the fuel injection system in a sports car, it drives us, it keeps us alive, setting objectives fires the mind.

It is no coincidence that Fauja Singh from Ilford in east London has lived beyond the age of 100. Fauja took up marathon running at the age of 89 being inspired to do so after watching televised coverage of the London Marathon. Fauja set himself the goal of learning how to run and then he ran one marathon after another, running a total of eight marathons between the ages of 89 and 101. At the age of 101 he decided his objective was not to retire but to shorten his running distance, to run a series of 5km and 10km races. I heard about Fauja in 2012, just as he reached the age of 101 and was in the throws of making his decision to only compete in shorter races (3). I have no idea if he is still running but if he is still alive I think he probably is.

People in Italy recognise the need to instill purpose in their life. *Tiriamo avanti,* literally, 'we pull ourselves forward', say the Italians when they talk about carrying on despite set backs encountered in their life. And I believe that sums up the relevance of life purpose and life goals. I believe we are beings of energy, that we are constructed in such a way that we are literally re-energised as soon as we set ourselves a goal.

Ronald Peters in his paper written upon the spontaneous remission of cancer, writes:

'FOLLOW YOUR EXCITEMENT AND FIND PASSION IN YOUR LIFE

Your immune system will work better if you find passion and happiness in your life. Following what excites you is your connection to your heart and to your spiritual nature (4).'

Scientists have discovered that those with purpose in their lives are less likely to suffer a stroke. During a four year assessment of adults over 50, all never having suffered from a stroke at the baseline of the assessment, it was determined, after adjustment for all other factors such as sex, age, race/ethnicity, marital status, education level, level of wealth, and functional status at baseline, that life purpose remained, *'significantly associated with a reduced likelihood of stroke (5)'.*

In 1946 an Austrian Psychiatrist, Victor Frankl wrote, *Man's Search for Meaning.* Victor Frankl survived a period of several years in a german concentration camp during WWII, whereas, tragically and as a result of great cruelty, very many died while still imprisoned. Victor Frankl lost his entire family in the holocaust. He as much as, or more so, than most human beings, would be justified in preparing a vitriolic and bitter account of his captivity, instead he wrote a deeply philosophical and selfless narrative, *Man's Search for Meaning* in the months after his release from the camp.

This work intended to inspire and instruct others, offers Victor Frankl's opinion on meaning within a life. On the relevance of life purpose he writes:

'Those who have a 'why' to live, can bear, with almost, any 'how'.

Victor Frankl considered that those who survived the concentration camps did so because they had a cause, mission, or unfulfilled desire in life to fulfill.

More explicitly he writes:

' Life is never made unbearable by circumstance, but only by lack of meaning and purpose'.

Victor Frankl did not consider that putting meaning in to your life, setting a target or a goal was simply a good idea.

Victor Frankl considered it was the responsiblity of every human being to imbue their own life with meaning if they wished to live fully and discover the full potential within themselves.

I wish to agree with him. I would say purpose of any kind, humble or grand, world changing or minimal is what is required.

If you are struggling to think of an activity, project or person that may give meaning to living, relax, perform the Ritual for several weeks and of itself a sense of purpose will arrive; a direction be revealed. I have absolutely no idea why this occurs but it happened to me and I believe there is something within the Ritual which changes thoughts and beliefs opening the door to activities and pursuits never previously considered.

I believe performing the Ritual leads a person to naturally incorporate in to their day new activities and people. It seems to be a natural adjunct of turning our attention inwards. Reflection upon the inner being unearths interests and creates directions never before considered. You will say I am biased in offering this opinion but I would say to all those who sense there is somthing lacking in their own lives, give the Ritual a go and see where turning inward takes you, monitor how your future life unfolds. Consider the number of passions and pursuits or new and interesting people you have incorporated within your life within one year or two of repetitive Ritual performance.

It is worth trying. It is a fact, tested scientifically by those working within the Rush University Medical Centre in Chicago that a sense of purpose in a life is even capable of changing the pathology of Alzheimer's disease.

Patricia Boyle and her colleagues from the Rush Alzheimer's Disease Centre studied 900 older adults, over an average of four years and a maximum of seven to assess whether having a purpose in life, (Purpose defined as living a life in which behaviour was guided by goals and intentions) which gave meaning to existence potentially protected the brain against harmful changes and plaques. The findings published in the Archives of General Psychiatry (6) determined that people who had a greater purpose in life had a substantially reduced risk of developing Alzheimer's disease, as well as a reduced risk, of mild cognitive impairment which is considered a forerunner to Alzheimers. Those who when questioned for the purpose of a psychological survey considered they had meaning and purpose in their life, whether through family, religion, pursuit of a passion such as an exercise regime or music were 2.4 times more likely to remain free of Alzheimers' as compared to other participants in the study unable to identify a pursuit activity or belief that gave meaning to their life. Lack of purpose being identified as one of the factors in health to increase the risk of onset of the disease.

Learn the lesson. If you are not, at the point at which you read this page, able to identify a pursuit passion or person that gives meaning to day to day existence it is time, I suggest, to re-think how you are living. Isolation, a lack of goals, of even the most modest type, is injurious.

Before I leave this chapter on the importance of each one of us finding purpose and so meaning in our own life I wish to direct my readers to a marvellous book dedicated to a philosophical and scientific explanation of the relevance of life purpose. It is the wonderful graphic novel, *On Purpose, Lessons In Life And Health From The Frog, The Dung Beetle, And Julia (7).*The author Victor J Strecher Phd, a Professor at the University of Michigan in the department of Public Health wrote *On Purpose* following the death of his 19 year old daughter Julia. The need for a purpose in life and how to attain purpose is examined from a scientific and philosophical perspective. This book is inspiring and illuminating and although produced out of the traumatic event of a daughter's death it is amusing and compassionate. I would recommend it to anyone searching for purpose in their own life. Victor Strecher provides us with a range of philosophical perspectives on finding purpose in life from the writings of Aldous Huxley, Simone de Beauvoir and many others, as well as dealing with the health benefits which result from seeking out purpose and meaning in our own existence.

In terms similar to Victor Frankl, Victor Strecher addresses the matter of self transcendence, of going beyond the ego to find life meaning and purpose by dedication of an individual life to something bigger than the self. This can be a person or a pursuit but self transcendence is recognised to be beneficial not only to finding contentment in life but also to promoting good health. Those with purpose function differently, their enzymes, including an important enzyme telomerase which protects the cap like structures on the end of our chromosones, is produced, in a different more efficient way, in a body driven by a mind directed by purpose. The consequence of the stimulation of the production of telomerase is that chromosones are less likely to fray or degenerate and the body is less likely to decline through the onset of disease. Result, what else but energised longevity!

CHAPTER FOURTEEN

OTHER SECRETS

I believe in my Ritual 100%. If there is one thing evident from a reading of this book it will be that fact. My Ritual is the singular most important aspect of my existence, but there are other aspects of my life that I consider I should not overlook as important to the good health, vitality and optimism that I am blessed with. The Ritual bears surprising fruit. It has become impossible for me, when analysing how I now live, to separate the things that came naturally to me before the Ritual began and the things to which the Ritual has given birth.

My present life is blessed by good fortune and good health. When I wake in the morning I am filled with joyful expectation about the day in front of me and I realise as I write this sentence how lucky I am and in what small percentage of similarly fated mankind that hopeful state of mind places me.

My Ritual helps. Re-engineering my thoughts has helped. I realise now I can be as happy and content as I wish to be. Happiness really is a state of mind. Without my Ritual I would not know that. The miracle of the Ritual is that it changes almost every aspect of an existence, changing priorities and outlook until an entirely new life is created.

I have no doubt the things I mention in this chapter have played their part in creating my present level of happiness and contentment.

HUMOUR

It is quite simply good for any person to see things from the lightest possible perspective. It is a truth we should all be acquainted with that it is not the situations life presents us with that matters but the manner in which we respond to the situations in which we are placed that counts. Most of the events of our lifetime, that engage our energy, or fuel our wrath or indignation, are, in the end, simply not that important. Months after even the most emotionally challenging matter has occurred we struggle to remember the precise details that enraged us, years later we cannot even relate the details clearly, the debris of the circumstance is ejected by our mind, and placed in the 'trivia' pile. I now see it is important to learn from our mistakes, battles and challenges. Do not let every day matters upset you, drain you, or steal your energy. Fill your brain with joy instead.

Laughter is good for human beings. Laughter reduces stress hormones and produces happy hormones, (endorphins). Laughing improves blood flow and can play an important role in reducing cardiovascular disease. Laughter even tones the abdominal muscles, making us look good as well as feel good. (1)

I believe we should purposely engage with humour. Watch comedy on TV or on 'You Tube'. Watch the best most humorous moments in movies. Do not watch the News or engage with world affairs day in and day out. A state of total ignorance is not desirable but total engagement with war, catastrophe, conflict, the rise and fall of stocks and shares, the economy, is really not necessary unless you are Home Secretary or your mission is politics.

Performing the Ritual has made it plain to me that everyone should turn towards the humour in their life. Engage with people who bring a little fun in to the situation, those who see the world in an entertaining way. Mixing with optimists makes you optimistic. Mixing with those who are negative, or constantly depressed, is like hanging a sack of ashes on your back and shutting the curtains on the sunshine.

The Ritual will alter your perspective just as it has mine. I believe within weeks of relaxing in to its meditative routine you will begin to see the world in a different way. I hope you enjoy the freshness in your outlook, the ease with which you begin to tackle living. Enjoyment is contagious, it will benefit those around you, and most importantly of all, finding the joy in life will benefit your health.

GO OUT FOR A WALK AND TAKE YOUR TIME

Troubles dissolve when we walk. Unresolved complexities resolve. Clarity comes. Try it. Walking is an act of meditation. The mind engages with the landscape and relaxes. All of the turbulence stress and indecision of our existence levels out in to a calm continuity of thought that provides the answers we may have been seeking for weeks. Arguments lose their bitterness; relationships regain their importance. The creative are inspired to design, plot, invent. The stressed are unwound, the sad restored, the angry calmed. All in the space of a walk, and it always works. Just keep going until the issue that takes you out walking is dealt with. There will always be enough miles.

The joy of walking is that it does not push us to our physical limits, steal our breath, exhaust us, as we aim at a new more demanding physical target. Walking does the opposite. It reminds us of our potential, illuminates our gifts, presents our lives in their best possible light, all while improving our health. It is for everyone, the super athlete and the armchair user. The slower you go and the further you go, the better it is for your health, (2), so do not worry about setting a fast pace. Just do it, get up from the couch and go for a walk. Your mind and your body will do the rest. Disconnect and immerse, all at the same time, enjoy the sunlight, the wind or the rain, the mud or the sand or the grass. With every step that you take you are walking your way to long life.

FILL UP YOUR DAY

In many respects it is like building your own school timetable. The good news is, your adult version of those blocked in squares on the calendar does not have to be the same every week, but it has to be full and it has to be colourful, and it has to be packed with interest.

Some may say, ' I wish', and suggest that they are not rich enough to create variety in their day.

Well I don't accept that. The big news is, and if you do not see it now the Ritual will make it evident, when you are retired, your wealth is in your health.

If you are pain and disease free, can walk, talk and enjoy the sunshine, you are a retirement billionaire!

Do something. That is what the Ritual will teach you. Engage with the world around you.

When you put your mind to it there are literally millions of things you can do with the rest of your life. It is not about money, it is about attitude. It costs nothing at all to stand up from the settee, turn off the TV and do something else.

It might just be walking, or it may be walking with a destination. It may be involving yourself in community projects or in art. It may be volunteering, after all you do not need money to be a volunteer, to help out in a shop or make a meal for someone confined to the house through age or isolation.

Get out of the house, meet people, meet them again. Drink tea, wine, or beer together, make a plan, go on an outing.

If you do not like that idea, stay inside. Sit down and consider what interests you. Perform the Ritual and when it is done spend an extra ten minutes communing with yourself. Think about the things you would really like to do, the hobbies you would like to pursue and take one step towards making your desires the reality of your life.

Do not wait until you are 105. Do not save up the following words to use when it really is too late. 'I always wanted to........but I never did'.

Do it now, not just one thing but dozens. Go dancing, go fishing, join the local history society and re-create the Battle of Bosworth on a Sunday afternoon. Bake a cake. Bake bread. Plant a flower. Take your junk to a car boot sale. Share your knowledge with somebody else; teach somebody something that you know.

As long as we are alive we have the capacity within us to be interested and interesting. Do not forget that. The world is a gigantic dome of engagement if we only take the time to open our eyes and see the millions of possibilities that are waiting for us, for our special gifts and qualities to lock in to what the Universe provides. If we believe in ourselves, in what we each have to offer, we will never be lonely because we will be taking part. It is what the Ritual teaches, and it is in the opening out of our life that we bring in good health.

HEALTH

It is all that matters.

Do all that you can every day to preserve the body and mind that you have.

CONTROL YOUR THOUGHTS

The Ritual involves a type of re- programming. It will come of its own accord. It is a side effect of performing the Ritual every day; the mind alters, whether as a result of neuroplasticity or another process I cannot say, but it does and the change is beneficial. It is almost as if the negative in every situation becomes less visible. The mind clings to or constructs from every incident the positive. An accumulation of positive thought, as we have seen, is life changing. The process is dynamic and enriching but it is not immediate. In the early stages of engaging with the Ritual negativity will still endeavour to make its appearance, to crowd the mind with worry anxiety, and irrelevancies, butting in to every thought we construct about every life decision to shadow it with bleakness, fear, insecurity and indecision.

The Ritual allows anyone, giving it the time, to see that it is quite simply time to kick negativity in to 'touch'. Time to take control of thought.

Several years in to performing the Ritual I can tell you that that can be done. We are more than our thoughts and we are master of them. What we think is up to us. We can let negativity run amok or we can keep it quiet, silence it by casting it out, thinking the converse of the worst. It will work, positivity will reign in your life and in your living if time and time again confronted with a negative thought you refuse to give it credence, laugh at it by summoning some invisible committee of the mind and shouting it down.

Negativity is powerful and consuming but it can be beaten back. Negative processing can literally be re-wired by an overwhelming refusal to see the downside. Eventually, through conditioning, the brain will choose the positive facts and aspects of a situation, each and every time. Even the most intransigent pessimist can I believe benefit from this technique.

Pessimists will of course say, 'it is not in their nature', or 'they are not pessimists but realists'. For the bleakly pessimistic or the depressive, controlling thought will be an uncomfortable struggle at first, like trying to put on an overcoat that does not fit. Stick with it. It works in the end, within weeks, months or years, depending upon your nature you will have changed forever the pattern of your thoughts and every aspect of your existence will have changed with your thinking. Not only that, the 'you' you discover beneath the debris of pessimism will be a being that is both inspiring and uplifting, and for whatever reason, whatever the magic within positivity, every cell in your body will be healthier and more resilient.

MINIMAL EXERCISING IS ALL IT TAKES

I used to be fanatical about pushing myself to the limits. Not now. Now as an inevitable consequence of the manner in which I commune with the body I have I have respect for my joints, for my muscles and sinews and ligaments and nerve endings. I am constantly aware of the machine of myself and I am constantly aware that, just as engineers employed by Ikea open and close a drawer to see how long the hinges will last, before the drawer wears out, so we must appreciate, we have joints that, just like hinges, can wear until they break.

I believe I have a finite number of movements within me, within the joints that I have and the muscles I contract and relax and the nerve endings I signal and message with, between the date of my lifetime and the date of my death. My Ritual I have no doubt will maximise my durability but however I look at it there is a point at which my body will wear out. Why bring that date forward by running successive marathons on one human set of knees or performing thousands of bench presses or lifts with weights until the body aches and complains?

I have no doubt over exercising is as bad for a body as not exercising at all. The fanatic who rises every day at 5.00am to be first in the pool at the gym, before completing circuits, to reach burn out time and time again, all in the course of a week, is not paying attention to the needs of the body. To the needs of the ego perhaps, but not to the needs of bone and tissue fibres constantly placed under stress.

The connection the Ritual forms between body and mind makes it impossible for the mind to accept the body should be pushed to extreme limits. It is as if the repetitive performance of a meditative Ritual causes the mania it is so easy to associate with exercise to subside. Preservation and maintenance of the body becomes the aim instead. Stretching replaces push ups, calm replaces the need for exertion to the point of collapse. Sport is still enjoyable, exercising to maintain fitness is still a goal of my life; it is just my approach that has changed.

I still enjoy all the sports that I did. I ski. I snowboard. I ride my bike. I kite surf. I simply set different goals or my mind does. I know when to stop, when to come off the water or away from the *piste*. In everything I do, I pay attention to myself, it is an inevitable consequence of 'listening in' and being, for the first time in my life, completely in tune with the body I possess. It is not a drawback, it is a gift, to realise and appreciate my humanness, not only my limits and vulnerabilities but my brilliance as a perfectly designed work of engineering that deserves admiration and respect.

DO WHAT YOU REALLY WANT TO WITH YOUR LIFE

It will make you live longer, in better health and with more 'spring in your step'. So many of us compromise, or even worse than that, do not engage so deeply with the decisions we make about the work that we do or the career that we establish, that we even realise a compromise has been made.

Usually our first big decision about what we want to do with our life is made at completely the wrong time, when we are teenagers, and completely unaware of what life holds or what our real gifts are.

Those choosing a profession are the worst offenders.

Following the conveyor belt of exam grades, university and work placements, many accountants, medics, bankers, barristers, dentists, and actuaries, end up in a channel, (or should I say rut), that carries them along for life, without once having the conversation they should have had, the one with their inner being and instinct; the one to be conducted in a room far away from academics and school teachers and career advisors and overbearing parents; the conversation with the self.

The good news is; it is never too late. Instinct builds and at whatever age you start to perform the Ritual instinct will be released. The long suppressed voice of inner desires and skills will become louder and louder until changes are made. I heard my self announce to my staff that the optical practice I had created was not somewhere I wanted to be, even though I had spent the best part of three decades testing patients, building up my reputation and my business. Within months of performing my Ritual I simply walked away. I shut the door on optics and began to build houses.

I didn't want to be an optician. What was I thinking of? I wanted to build, architecturally pleasing houses, in the style of the English vernacular. Barge board and perfect proportion, houses that stood out and were admired, houses that would leave a footprint of my own existence upon the planet. I should have been building all of my life.

I should by now have created a model village, my own, *Blaize Hamlet*, but I had failed to listen to myself. The Ritual changed all that. Now I know I am living as I was intended to live. I am utilising the gifts that I have and I am giving vent to my creativity and passion and as a consequence I am a happy and contented man.

Anyone reading this, who is in the wrong occupation, will sense that within his or herself. It is back to the overcoat that does not fit. Performing the Ritual will ensure the overcoat is set aside and another coat chosen.

Try it.

Whatever age you are now trust me, it is not too late to begin. Re-train. Take another degree, begin an apprenticeship. Age is changing, society is changing. Second careers will soon be as likely as was retiring age 55, save retiring at 55 is now a pointless thing to do.

So get the decision right this time. Tune in to the being you are. Have the conversation with yourself you have postponed all of your life. You have decades left to live, make sure you live them well with contented organs and cells. Make every vein and artery of yourself perform to its full potential as you run with the current of your life instead of against it. Do what you really want to do with your existence and you will be here for a very long time.

THERE IS NO VALUE IN OSTENTATION

Realise that and you will be happier. It is not necessary to live in the biggest house, to have the biggest most expensive car. It is not necessary to have fine jewels or gold watches or tailored suits or shoes costing hundreds and hundreds of pounds. There is no value in ostentation; the value is in the self, in the cells of your being and the flesh on your back; in individual intelligence and spirit and humanness.

The Ritual makes that evident. And let me make it clear. I do not propose that all those who dedicate themselves to the Ritual need to live naked without possessions in a self imposed ascetism. I do not believe that for one minute. I do believe however that within weeks or months of performing the Ritual the performer will come to see the value inside him or herself. Value will be 'brought home to roost', and will rest internally rather than be represented by a pile of external possessions. Accumulating possessions will become less necessary.

For whatever reason the Ritual causes a shift in perspective that allows the performer of this simple therapeutic programme to recognise their own internal worth. Once this fountain of real incalculable wealth is connected with, the prize in ostentation loses its glitter.

I downsized my house, gave away all the furniture that would not fit inside my smaller home. I built a walled garden around my considerably reduced patch of ground and I designed a small but perfect garden that has become one of the joys of my life. I have lived in mansions surrounded by acres of land but I have never felt the joy in the experience I feel now when I place myself in the middle of my flowers, on a low lounger, in the shade of an umbrella. I notice colour, form, and shape. I perform my Ritual and I feel a deep sense of contentment.

I drive a builder's truck instead of a top of the range sportscar. I will never be able to explain it but the Ritual has made me see the value in simplicity and the pointlessness of trying to give a value to our life by spending vast sums of money on possessions acquired to impress. We are already impressive, each one of us. The Ritual reveals that fact. Life is easier and so much less complicated once we realise our value is inside us and not in the car on our driveway.

LOVE YOURSELF

If you do not already the Ritual will cause you to. If you do not love yourself you cannot love anyone else. It is one of the biggest lessons the Ritual delivers, we must connect with and love the being that we are if we are to live as we are intended to. I have said before and I will say it again, all the compassion we have in our heart that we are ready to bestow upon others we must also bestow upon our own self. Love is the most powerful emotion we possess. If every day, we do not, 'give ourselves a break', forgive our weaknesses, recognise our individual strengths and acknowledge how great we truly are, the potential we possess, we do not fully live.

Try it now.

Let the emotion I talk about fill every cell of your body.

Allow your own mind to hold and release, the enrichment of love and compassion, that you will, an untold number of times in your life, have bestowed upon others, rush from your mind, along every vein and artery you possess, to not only your heart, but in to every organ and structure you consist of.

It feels good doesn't it? It feels, don't you agree, like a release? And it is, from all the decay and devastation of age. Become practised at showering love upon yourself, it is the most powerful gift you possess. It will renew you, and that is why the Ritual was created.

ENDNOTES

CHAPTER ONE

1. Report by Ellen Warner MD. Pub. Can Med Assoc. J. Vol 128. May 1983.
2. John Robbins *Healthy at 100. Ballantine Books. Copyright John Robbins 2006.*

CHAPTER TWO

1. J.A.M.A December 24th 1955.1602.The Powerful Placebo. Henry K.Beecher. M.D Boston
2. Faith Brynie Phd on her web page Brain Sense and in her book of the same name, Brain Sense, (Amazon 2009) documents a number of placebo experiments reporting a variation of success rates for placebos ranging from 15% to 72%. Placebo success varying with the number of physician visits a patient receives and duration of treatment.
3. Daniel E Moerman Phd and Wayne B Jonas. MD. Ann Intern Med.2002;136;471-476
4. See paper prepared by Anne Harrington for the 2002 symposium, entitled; 'Seeing' the Placebo Effect; historical legacies and present opportunities.
5. Both trials demonstrating the impact of a physician's message are referred to by Daniel Moerman in his paper *Deconstructing the Placebo Effect and Finding the Meaning Response. P.472*
6. Listening to Prozac but Hearing Placebo: A Meta Analysis of Antidepressant Medication. Kirsch/Sapirstein. Prevention&Treatment. Volume1. Article 0002a. 26/6/1998.
7. Placebo Therapy of benign prostatic hyperplasia: a 25 month study. Canadian PROSPECT Study Group.Br.J.Urol.1998. Mar,81(3);383-7.
8. Fabrizio Benedetti et al. Journal of Neuropsychopharmacology. Jan 2011;36(1):339-354.Published online June 30, 2010.
9. Effects of Expectation on Placebo Induced Dopamine Release in Parkinson's Disease.Arch Gen Psychiatry.Vol.67 (No 8) August 2010

10. Effects of Perceived Treatment on Quality of Life and Medical Outcomes in a Double-blind Placebo Surgery Trial
11. Reported in the New England Journal of Medicine 1959.
12. Arthroscopic Treatment of Osteoarthritis of the Knee: A Prospective, Randomized, Placebo-Controlled Trial: Results of a Pilot Study. Am. J. Sports Medicine. Jan 1996 (24)28-34
13. Frank & Frank 1991
14. Active Albuterol or Placebo, Sham Acupuncture or No Intervention in Asthma. Michael E Wechsler et al. N.Eng J Med.2011;365;119-126. July 14th 2011

CHAPTER THREE

1 Ibid. Chapter 2. Endnote 9
2 Double Blind versus deceptive administration of a placebo. Kirch.I Weixel. LJ. Journal of Behavioural Neuroscience 1988:102(2);319---323
3 Ibid. Chapter 2. Endnote 6
4 Explanatory mechanisms for placebo effects: cognition, personality and social learning. A paper prepared by Richard Bootzin for the symposium on placebo. Ibid Chapter 2. Endnote 4
5 Ibid.Chapter 2. Endnote 3.
6 Placebo Studies and Ritual Theory: a comparative analysis of Navajo, acupuncture and biomedical healing. Ted J. Kaptchuk. Philos Trans R Soc Lond B Biol Sci June 27 2011;366 (1572);1849---1858
7 This email is referred to in the Harvard Magazine. Online Issue March---April 2013. P4.

CHAPTER FOUR

1 Big Pharma: How the World's Biggest Drug Companies Control Illness.2006 by British Journalist Jacky Law. See also Bad Pharma (2012) Ben Goldacre
2 Journal of Autonomic Neuroscience. Vol. 164. Issues 1---2. 28th October 2011. P 62---66. Organ Specificity of placebo effects on blood pressure. K.Meissner. D.Ziep.
3 Journal of Orthopaedic Nursing. July/Aug 2005---Vol24.Issue4. p259--- 269.Energy Healing. A Complementary Therapy for Orthopaedic and Other Conditions. DNucci, Ellen M

4   Mia Hansson reporting for the Guardian: NHS recognition
     mindfulness meditation is good for depression. Reported 26th
     February 2013.

5   Reported on Mental Health Foundation Website.Source ICM
     Survey of 250 GP's. June 2009.

6   Alterations in Brain and Immune Function Produced by
     Mindfulness--- Meditation. Richard J Davidson Phd. Jon
     Kabat---Zinn, Phd. Et al Collaboration between Dept. of
     Psychology University of Wisconsin, Dept of Medicine,
     University of Massachussetts Dept of Medicine &
     Microbiology, University of Wisconsin. Dept of History of
     Science, Harvard University. Clinics Centre of Wisconsin,
     Madison Wisconsin. Dept of Oral Biology, Ohio State
     University.

7   Psychology Today: Published on the 22nd May 2013. Rebecca
     Gladding MD identifies the areas of the brain affected by
     meditation. She describes changes to neural pathways,
     produced through meditation, in and between the lateral
     prefrontal cortex; the medial prefrontal cortex; the insula and
     the Amydala.

8   Harvard Gazette:21.01.11 Article, 'Eight Weeks to a better
     Brain'. Reporting on the effects of Sarah Lazar's study in to
     the benefits of meditation upon the brain. Sarah Lazar is an
     instructor in Psychology in the Harvard Medical School.

9   Eliss Epel findings reported in the New Scientist. Issue 30th
     August 2011 in an article Heal Thyself: Meditate.

10   As reported on Helpguide. Org, produced in collaboration with
     Harvard Medical Publications and the Harvard Medical School.
     Article: The Benefits of Mindfulness Practices for Improving
     Emotional and Physical Well Being.

11   Akira Otani. University of Maryland Counseling Centre.
     Eastern Meditative Techniques and Hypnosis: A New
     Synthesis. American Journal of Clinical Hypnosis (46) 2nd
     October 2003.See Table 1. Comparison of Western v Eastern
     Healing Paradigms.

12   Motor Imagery in Physical Therapist Practice. Journal of
     Physical Therapy July 2007: Vol 87 no 7 942---953

13   A clinical study of visualisation on depressed white blood cell
     count in medical patients. PMID 10932336. Donaldson VW.

Center For Stress Management, Carrboro, North Carolina 27510 USA.

14   Mind Over Matter: Mental Training Increases Physical Strength. Erin M Shackell and Lionel G Standing. Bishops University Canada. .North American Journal of Psychology. 2007.Vol 9. No 1.

15   The Effects of Guided Imagery on the Immune System: A Critical Review. Trakhtenbery EC. Institute of Transpersonal Psychology, Palo Alto, California 94303 USA

16   Effects Among Healthy Subjects of the Duration of Regularly Practising a Guided Imagery Program. Watanabe E. et al. Department of Health Promotion and Human Behaviour Kyoto University Graduate School of Public Health

17   The sculpture depicted on the cover of the Ritual is an original art work by of Simon Watson (copyright reserved), an artist living and working in Burton On Trent in Staffordshire. For further examples of his work see his website. www.simonwatsonart.co.uk

CHAPTER SEVEN

1   See John Robbins study of the Abkhasia: Ancients of the Caucasus in *Healthy at 100*. 2007 Ballantine Books New York

2   Molecules of Emotion. Pg 286 -287. Candace B. Pert. Ph.D. Published by Simon&Schuster 1998. Pocket Books Edition. 1999.

3   The pituitary gland has been called the 'conductor of the endocrine orchestra'. The Oxford Companion to the Body 2001. Colin Blakemore and Sheila Jennett.

   I believe my pituitary shower also stimulates the hypothalamus and is beneficial in enhancing circulation of cerebro spinal fluid.

CHAPTER TEN

1   Neurobiological Mechanisms of the Placebo Effect. Fabrizio Benedetti et al. The Journal of Neuroscience 9.11.2005. 25 (45);10390---10402

2   Ibid. (8)CH 2.

3   The Opposite Effects of the Opiate Antagonist Naloxone
     and the Cholecystokinin Antagonist Proglumide or Placebo
     Analgesia. Fabrizio Benedetti. Pain. Vol 64. Issue 3; 535---
     543. Conscious Expectation and Unconscious Conditioning in
     Analgesic, Motor and Hormonal Placebo/Nocebo Responses.
     Benedetti Pollo et al. The Journal of Neuroscience May 15
     2003;23 (10);4315---4323

4   Harvard Magazine ; March---April 2013 Online Edition p.4

5   Response Expectancies In Placebo Analgesia and their Clinical
     Relevance. Pollo A, Amanzio M, et al. Pain. 2001. Jul. 93; 77--
     -84

6   Snake Oil Science. R Barker Bausell 2007 Oxford University
     Press.

7   Placebo---Responsive Parkinson Patients show decreased
     activity in Single Neurons of the Sub---Thalamic Nucleus.
     Benedetti, Colloca et al. Journal of Nature Neuroscience 7.587-
     --588 (2004)

8   Brain Activity Associated with Expectancy---Enhanced
     PlaceboAnalgesia as Measured by Functional Magnetic
     Resonance Imaging. Kong, Gollub et al. The Journal of
     Neuroscience, 11th January 2006;26(2);381---388 A Functional
     Magnetic Resonance Imaging Study on the Neural Mechanisms
     of Hyperalgesic Nocebo Effect. Kong, Gollub et al. The
     Journal of Neuroscience. December 3rd 2008; 28(49);13354---
     13362

9   Stewart Wolf MD. Psychiatrist and Consultant Neurologist,
     often referred to as 'the father of psychosomatic medicine'.
     Wolf S: Effects of Suggestion and Conditioning on the Action
     of Chemical Agents In Human Subjects: The Pharmacology of
     Placebos. Journal of Clinical Investigation. 1950 Jan. 29(1);
     100---109

10   Lynoe N. Placebo is not always effective against nocebo
     bacilli. The Body –Mind Inter---play still Wrapped in Mystery.
     Läkartidningen 2005. Sep 19---25;102(38);2627---8

11   Meditaton Research; Monthly Archives Mar 2014. Meditation
     and Neuroplasticity: Five Key Articles

12   Dr David Hamiliton. You Tube Interview Dr David Hamilton
     University of Strathclyde: Science Proves That Our Thoughts
     Count

13   Navigation---Related Structural change in the Hippocampi of taxi drivers. Maguire E,Gadian D et al. PNAS Vol 97.No8.4398---4403

14   Sea Gypsies of Asia Boast 'incredible' Underwater Vision. Natural Geographic online. Article by Brian Handwerk May14th 2004 reporting on the study by Anna Gislen of the Moken people.

15   Brain Plasticity and Stroke Rehabilitation. The Willis Lecture. Barbro B Johnansson. Stroke 2000 Jan; 31(1): 223---30

16   The Mind and the Brain: Neuroplasticity and the Power of Mental Force. Schwartz, Jeffrey et al. Regan Books. Harper Collins Publisher (2002)

17   The Harvard Piano Study reported in Time Magazine 19th January 2007.

18   The Biology of Belief. Bruce H. Lipton Phd. Hay House Publications 2008

19   Changes in Prostate Gene Expression In Men Undergoing An Intensive Nutrition and Lifestyle Intervention. Ornish D et al. Proc Natl. Acad Sci USA. 2008 June 17;105(24);8369---74

20   Candace Pert *Molecules of Emotion*--- Why You Feel The Way You Feel. Pocket Books 1999; An imprint of Simon&Schuster Inc.

21   Ibid. p286

22   Ibid. p273

23   Ibid. p252

24   Philosophical Transactions of the Royal Society B. Biological Sciences:Spirituality: An Overlooked Predictor of Placebo Effects 16th May 2011

25   Enhancement of Cancer Chemotherapy by the Pineal Hormone Melatonin and its relation with the Psychospiritual Status of Cancer Patients. Messina.Lissoni et al 2010.

26   A Controlled Trial of Arthroscopic Surgery for Osteoarthritis of the Knee. J Bruce Moseley, MD, et al. N Eng J Med 2002;347;81---88

27   A Randomized Trial of Vertebroplasty for Painful Osteoporotic Vertebral Fractures. Buchbinder et al and Kalmes et al. NEJM 2009:361(6):557---568 and 569---579

28   Online report of Dr Chris Beedie placebo trial. Aberystwyth University Web Page 17th February 2014

29   Ted Kaptchuk: Placebo Studies and Ritual Theory: a
      comparative analysis of Navajo, Acupuncture and Bio Medical
      healing. Philosophical Transactions of the Royal Society B.
      Biological Sciences. Published 16th May 2011.
30   Ibid
31   Ibid
32   The Journal of Mind Body Regulation. Examining a Powerful
      Healing Effect through a Cultural Lens and finding Meaning.
      Daniel Moerman Phd. 63 MBR Vol 1. Issue 2.

CHAPTER ELEVEN

1   B.L Fredrickson. The Broaden and Build Theory of Positive
      Emotions. Department of Psychology. The University of
      Michigan. Published Online 17th August 2004
2   Psychological Resilience and Positive Emotional Granularity:
      Examining the Benefits of Positive Emotions on Coping and
      Health. Tugade et al; J. Pers. 2004 Dec 72 (6) 1161-1190.
3   Annals of Behavioural Medicine. Vol 39.p 4.
4   Journal of Psychosomatic Medicine. Vol70. P 741.
5   Understanding Centenarians Psychosocial Dynamics and Their
      Contributions to Health and Quality of Life. Poon et al. Current
      Gerontology and Geriatrics Research, Volume 2010.
6   Ed Diener et al. 'Happy People Live Longer: Subjective
      Well-Being Contributes to Health and Longevity'. Journal of
      Applied Psychology. Health and Well Being. Vol 3. Issue 1.
      March 2011.
7   Anthony. D.Ong Department of Human Development, G77
      Martha Van Rensselaer Hall, Cornell University, Ithaca, NY:
      Pathways Linking Positive Emotion and Health In Later Life.
      Current Directions in Psychological Science December 2010.
      Vol 19. No 6 358-362.

CHAPTER TWELVE

1   Greg Bradden. Writer. Belief Code 24A.
2   International Agency For Research On Cancer. Press release
      No 223. 12th Dec. 2013.
3   World Health Organisation. Factsheet No 317.

4   Office of National Statistics. Register of Medical Cause of
     Death 2012.
5   In 2014 after 60 years of contrary advice Dr James di
     Nicolantonio a leading cardiovascular research scientist at
     the Mid America Heart Institute published the results of his
     research which he said demonstrated that advice given over
     the last 60 years as to the relevance of a diet low in saturated
     fats to the prevention of heart disease was, ' deeply flawed'. Dr
     Nicolantonio identifies instead, 'sugar' as the culprit and wants
     warnings to be given as to the amount of sugar that should be
     consumed on a daily basis.
6   Statistics from the US Centre for Disease Control. Research
     Date 23.12. 2013
7   The cases of Serge Perrin and Delizia Cirolli are documented
     in the account of the Lourdes Medical Bureau provided on
     Wikipedia. Facts extracted 31.10.13
8   Breznitz. Study of Fighter Pilots in WW11.
9   Ronald Peters, MD, MPH from the Mind Body Medicine
     Center 13951 N. Scottsdale, Suite 100. Scottsdale, Arizona
     85254
10   Ibid p.8

CHAPTER THIRTEEN

1   John Robbins founder of EarthSave International (a non profit
     organization dedicated to healthy food choices, preservation of
     the environment and a more compassionate world). Healthy at
     100. Ballantine Books. 2007.
2   Ibid p57.
3   BBC London news report; 22.11.2012.
4   Ronald Peters MD, MPH Mind Body Medicine Center
     Scottsdale Arizona. Spontaneous Remission of Cancer.
5   Journal of Psychosomatic Research. 'Purpose in life and
     reduced incidence of stroke in older adults: 'The Health and
     Retirement Study'. 1.03.2013.
6   Archives of General Psychiatry Issue March 2010.
7   *On Purpose: Lessons In Life and Health from The Frog, The
     Dung Beetle and Julia.* Available on Amazon and In Paperback.
     Author Victor J. Strecher

CHAPTER FOURTEEN

1   Laughology. Improve Your Life With the Science of Laughter. Professor William Fry from Stanford University. USA. Professor Fry dubs laughing as 'internal jogging' because of the effect it has upon the muscles of the body.

2   A Norwegian Study. 'Minimal Intensity Physical Activity (Standing and Walking) of Longer Duration Improves Insulin Action and Plasma Lipids More Than Shorter Periods of Moderate to Vigorous Exercise (Cycling) in Sedantary Subjects When Energy Expenditure is Comparable. Published. 13.02.13. Plos One. DOI:10.1371/Journal.pone.0055542. Hans. H.E.M Savelberg et al. This study demonstrated long periods of four hour slow walking and two hours standing per day were better for the body in terms of over all physiological results than one hour of high intensity cycling.